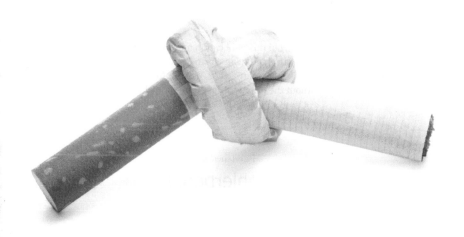

Where there is a will, there is a way.

14 & Out

by Sean David Cohen

ISBN 978-1-9401922-3-9

Published by

◤ **köehlerbooks**™

210 60th Street
Virginia Beach, VA 23451
212-574-7939
www.koehlerbooks.com

Publisher
John Köehler

Executive Editor
Joe Coccaro

Author's Note

I have taken careful measures to ensure the accuracy and usefulness of the information in this book, but I am not, nor do I in any way pretend to be, a medical expert or medically trained. I am, like most of you, a layman. But I am also a journalist trained to find facts, observe behavior and do research.

Helping people avoid harmful chemicals and live healthier has been my passion and professional field of expertise. Yet please understand that *14 & Out* is a self-help book that is more about behavior modification, motivation and awareness. It is not a treatise on chemistry and the physiology of contracting and treating cancer or other smoking-related ailments. But I am not shy about strongly advocating good nutrition and health as a way to combat cigarette addiction and improve your quality of life.

This stop-smoking guide is grounded in research but does not constitute medical advice and should not be used as a substitute for seeing a licensed physician, nutritionist or medical advisor if you are ill or think you might be. If this book inspires you to quit smoking or, in even a small way, improves your health, vitality and happiness, it will have served its purpose.

Dedicated to my Grandfather Sol,

who was a two-pack a day smoker and died from it.

Had we only known then what we know now.

14 & OUT

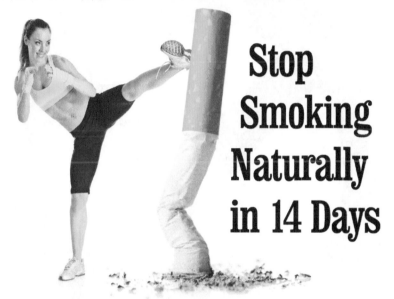

Stop Smoking Naturally in 14 Days

A Step-by-Step Guide to Freedom and Health

Sean David Cohen

Author of *Don't Eat Cancer*

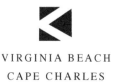

VIRGINIA BEACH
CAPE CHARLES

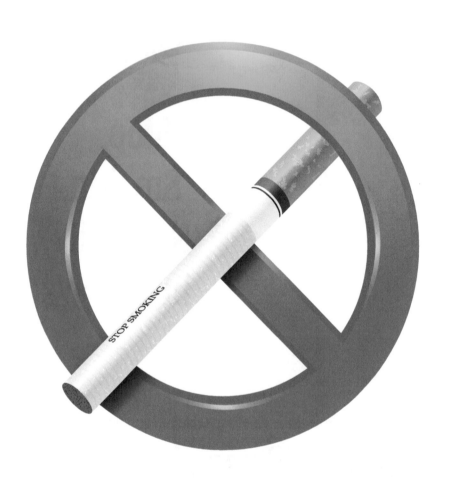

Foreword

Cigarettes and the chemicals that comprise them are manufactured and sold at high profit by some of the most powerful corporations in the world. That makes it all the more strange that many of today's most popular treatments for cigarette addiction are also chemicals manufactured and sold at high profit by a few of the other most powerful corporations in the world. Cigarette addiction treatment, it seems, often involves little more than the transfer of substance addiction from one corporation (tobacco companies) to another (drug companies). Something is fundamentally wrong with this approach.

14 & Out offers readers a new approach to quitting the smoking habit for good—an approach that frees you from all corporation chemicals and their physiological addictions. It does this by addressing smoking addiction with a multi-layered approach, reforming smoking behaviors, detoxifying the body from chemicals that promote addiction, and supporting the body's healthy functioning with a sound nutritional approach that works with the brain's natural chemistry to break addictions at a molecular level.

While no strategy works for everyone, the *14 & Out* approach has the unique advantage of addressing smoking addiction from a holistic point of view (i.e., taking into account the whole person who is addicted, including their behaviors and habits, nutritional foundation, physiology and more). Perhaps that's why it works so well for those who truly apply it.

With this system, people who really wish to quit smoking now have a road map to success that really works. It's not a chemical trick nor a temporary Band-Aid. It's a lifelong solution to reclaiming your health, your discretionary income and possibly even saving your own life.

That's why I urge you to not merely read this book, but to actually put it into action. Let Sean Cohen coach you on the path toward addiction freedom that countless others before you have already achieved.

In the near future, after you've beat the smoking addiction, you'll look back at your decision today and thank yourself for having the courage and foresight to follow a new journey that leads to personal success.

Congratulate yourself on your willingness to invest the time in allowing this book to guide you on that pathway to personal health freedom. I am confident it will be the best investment of time and effort you'll ever make.

–Mike Adams, The Health Ranger
  Founder of NaturalNews.com and director of
  the Natural News Forensic Food Laboratory
  (FoodInvestigations.com)

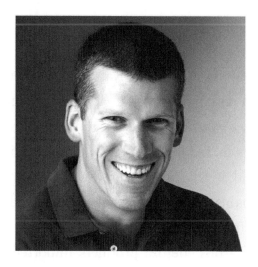

About the Foreword Author: Mike Adams (aka the "Health Ranger") is the founding editor of NaturalNews.com, the Internet's number one natural health news website, now reaching seven million unique readers a month.

With a background in science and software technology, Adams is the original founder of the e-mail newsletter technology company known as Arial Software. Using his technical experience combined with his love for natural health, Adams developed and deployed the content management system currently driving NaturalNews.com. He also engineered the high-level statistical algorithms that power SCIENCE.naturalnews.com, a massive research resource now featuring over ten million scientific studies.

In addition to being the co-star of the popular Gaiam TV series called *Secrets to Health*, Adams is also the (non-paid) executive director of the non-profit Consumer Wellness Center (CWC), an organization that redirects one hundred percent of its donations to grant programs that teach children and women how to grow their own food or vastly improve their nutrition.

In 2013, Adams created the Natural News Forensic Food Laboratory, a research lab that analyzes common foods and supplements, reporting the results to the public. He is well known for his incredibly popular consumer activism video blowing the lid on fake blueberries used throughout the food supply. He has also exposed "strange fibers" found in Chicken McNuggets, fake academic credentials of so-called health "gurus," dangerous "detox" products imported as battery acid and sold for oral consumption, fake acai berry scams, the California raw milk raids, the vaccine research fraud revealed by industry whistle-blowers and many other topics.

Adams has also helped defend the rights of home gardeners and protect the medical freedom rights of parents. Adams is widely recognized to have made a remarkable global impact on issues like genetically modified organisms (GMOs), vaccines, nutrition therapies and human consciousness.

In addition to his activism, Adams is an accomplished musician who has released ten popular songs covering a variety of activism topics.

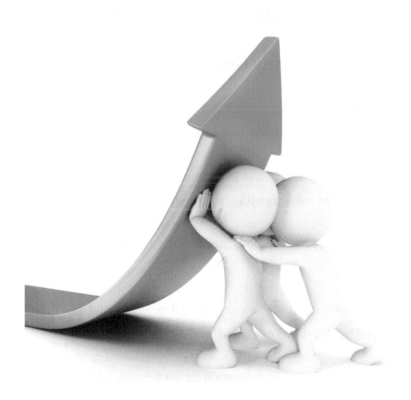

Table of Contents

Part I: The Daily Guide (pp 23 – 50)

❏ Learn why *14 & Out* has proven results and a high-success ratio for getting smokers to stop smoking forever.

❏ Understand why ninety-five percent of smokers who quit without help go back to smoking within six months.

❏ Know exactly what the body needs daily to kill the cravings of nicotine.

❏ Straight talk on central nervous system deficiencies and how to feel "normal" and "relaxed or excited" without nicotine.

❏ Whether you smoke for relaxation or confidence, this program is designed for you. Take the simple steps and follow the "yellow brick road" to good health.

❏ Whether you smoke a pack a day, two packs a day, or even more, you can still quit within two weeks.

❏ Even if you've been smoking for twenty years, these strategies apply to you.

Part II: What Really Goes Up In Smoke? (pp 51 - 70)

❑ Find out why cigarettes burn so hot, so evenly, and never go out in heavy wind and how this heightens the addiction.

❑ Find out how and why the nicotine potency you're getting is thirty-five times stronger than you think.

❑ Get the inside scoop on which household chemicals are used to manufacture a cigarette in order to keep you hooked.

❑ Understand why it's the chemicals in cigarettes more than the nicotine that's fueling the habit and the vicious cycle.

❑ Know how Marlboro almost put all other brands out of business and how that plays into premium brands hooking more smokers.

❑ Learn how you can wake up in the morning without coughing or needing a cigarette.

Part III: Dangerous Alternatives (pp 71 - 84)

❑ Learn why the pills fail so many smokers who try them.

❑ Understand the risks of taking pharmaceuticals like Chantix and Zyban.

❑ Know why the nicotine patch and nicotine gum are far cries from real help.

❑ Understand why hypnotherapy and electronic cigs are rarely the answer.

Part IV: Nutrition, The Only Alternative (pp 85 - 95)

❑ Get knowledge of proper nutrients, antioxidants, herbs and supplements recommended by highly regarded professionals who understand the process of quitting smoking.

❑ Say goodbye to nervousness, anxiety, depression, sleeplessness, and a host of others symptoms of smokers who stop smoking—this course is one hundred percent natural and organic.

❑ Take a twenty-question pretest to test your knowledge of your habit, and then hear the answers and explanations that reveal all the secrets of how to stop smoking.

Part V: The "New You" Does Great Things! (pp 96 - 118)

❑ Understand how breathing patterns changed when you became a smoker and how you can get back to having healthy lungs and a healthy heart.

❑ Learn how to replace bad habits with good, natural, healthy ones that keep you from ever being a smoker again.

❑ As a nonsmoker, you won't be a burden for those around you, including the ones you love most.

❑ You will save thousands of dollars and have new energy for the extra-curricular activities you enjoy.

❑ The knowledge you gain from *14 & Out* is yours forever; nobody can steal it, and you can't lend it out and forget to get it back!

Tests, Resources, Testimonials (pp 119 - 135)

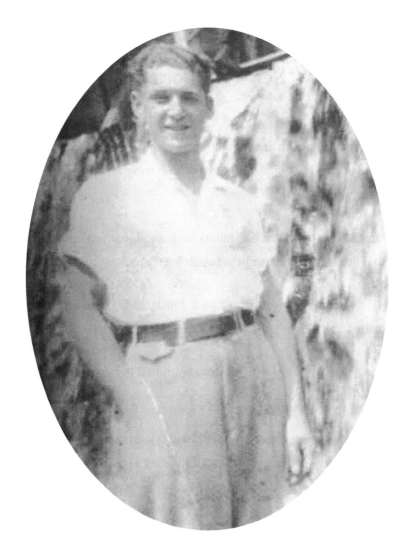

Sol Gross
1911—1975

My Inspiration

As a six-year old boy, I remember my Grandfather Sol skipping rope in the garage. I didn't realize it would be the last time I ever saw him. I've been told that he never admitted that his cancer came from smoking. Even his doctor, who was his best friend, smoked. My mother and I watched my grandfather smoke himself to death. I remember him jumping rope in our garage a couple of months before it got really bad. I was so impressed. He had the will to live, so what happened? Lung cancer ate him down to the bone.

My grandfather was not a tall man, only about five foot six inches, but my mom said he weighed only eighty-eight pounds when he died, compared to about one hundred and forty before the cancer. The doctor told him at one point that if he kept smoking, he would surely die within two years. He couldn't quit. This was in the early 1970s, when Big Tobacco had already started using ammonia to heighten the addiction. Though my grandfather loved his family and his life, he couldn't quit because he didn't know how to quit.

I won't let this happen to you. For every person I get to

quit smoking, my grandfather's soul, his life, is redeemed a little bit more. It is my motivation to create this all-natural program, teach it, and keep it up to date and write about it as long as I live.

Though I smoked cigarettes and drank alcohol in college, I thought of Grandfather Sol and what happened to him, and I quit the toxic habits before they could get the best of me. And though I had my fair share of fast food and "simple" pleasures, I am currently an organic vegetarian who remains committed to maintaining perfect health and peace of mind. I am a student for life, focused on learning and perfecting my writing to best share this evolving process.

When I went to college to study journalism at the University of Georgia in 1986, and then returned to UGA in 1994 to get my master's degree in education, I started picking up books about chemicals not only in cigarettes, but in food, candy, gum, cosmetics, you name it. I wanted to put all of my research to good use and hopefully prevent people from ever having to go through the nightmare of cancer.

For years, I studied about the chemicals in cigarettes and how they affect the body. A forthcoming book of mine called *Don't Eat Cancer* contains four chapters about all the hidden secrets about cigarettes that Big Tobacco does not want you to know or understand. During my research I couldn't believe everything I was reading and realizing. I wanted to put this information to use, so I began teaching a one-hour class for free at public libraries on how to quit smoking.

Smokers attending the sessions ask me a lot of poignant questions, some of which I don't always have the answers

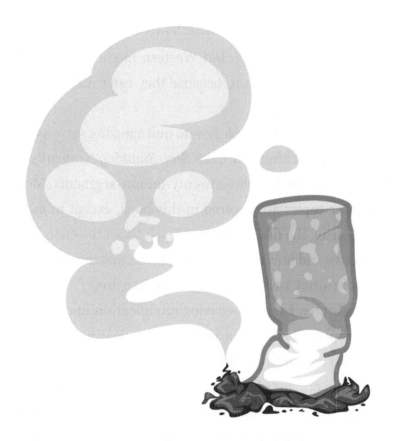

to right on the spot. However, most of the questions I have heard before or researched those topics, and the answers astound them and always make the class more interesting and exciting for everyone. If I don't have the answer to a question, we discuss it, figure out the common sense approach to dealing with it and we move on. Quitting smoking is not a perfect science, but I have thoroughly researched every stop-smoking method out there, and the best chance you have to stop smoking forever is *14 & Out*.

Most of my research is ongoing, so I always keep my eyes open for new gimmicks, new ways Big Tobacco tries to hook smokers and keep them hooked, and I often dispel the myths associated with natural remedies. Trust me, Mother Nature has a cure for everything, but Western medicine does not want you to know about it, because they can't make money off you if you're healthy.

My years teaching people how to quit smoking serve as the foundation for writing *14 & Out—Stop Smoking Naturally In 14 Days*. The class has three twenty-minute segments. Most of the same topics are covered in this book, except in more depth. During the first segment, I teach about the chemicals in cigarettes and how they bring you down, making you crave relief from what I term "the cigarette hangover." The next twenty minutes I teach behavior modification and exactly how to replace bad habits with healthy routines. For the final twenty minutes, I share the nutrition and supplements that end the cravings for cigarettes and replenish a severely damaged digestive and breathing system. This section comprises a crucial list of organic and natural food, beverages and herbs that I have gathered from some of the world's leading nutrition experts and doctors, including Mike Adams, founder and editor of NaturalNews.com, the world's leading health news website. I have been a frequent contributor to Mike's website and a student of his teachings. I have also had the pleasure of learning from David Wolfe, one of the world's leading nutritionists, herbalists and world travelers. I am also fortunate to have in-depth discussions about *14 & Out* and related nutrition with Dr. Richard DiCenso, author of *Beyond Medicine*.

I have also interviewed and consulted with doctors, nurses, X-ray technicians, physicians' assistants, nutritionists,

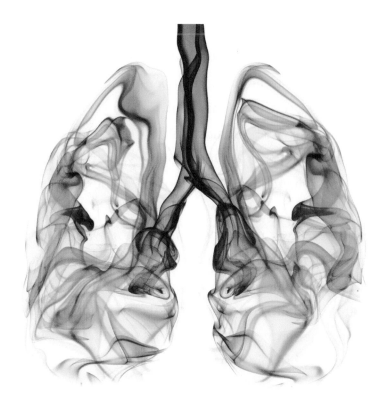

naturopathic physicians, raw food experts, cooks, athletes, mixed martial arts experts, massage therapists, chiropractors, scientists, surgeons, gastroenterologists, hundreds of smokers, ex-smokers and people who have tried other cessation programs. *14 & Out* was born from their collective wisdom.

The world is filled with half-truths and flat-out misinformation when it comes to health and health products, so I am going to be very direct, even blunt, with my assessments of Big Tobacco and reasons why cigarettes are so addictive. It's important to understand the context for addiction. So you will find in these pages a close examination of the ingredients in cigarettes, the behavior of some cigarette manufacturers and a layman's explanation of the consequences of smoking these products. There are also discussions on eating well and a resource guide to help you with your own research. I also include a Q&A section in this book to help smokers quickly get some answers to their most burning questions.

I call my steps *14 & Out* because you are weaned off nicotine and the total habit of smoking in fourteen days, or sometimes less.

Quite simply, this method is for those who have tried other ways to quit and have had no luck. For most people, the pills, the patch, the gum and e-cigarettes do nothing but delay an inevitable return to the deadly addiction of cigarette smoking. The devices and substances are alternatives, not a panacea for breaking an addiction. They keep your body dependent.

Some people quit cold turkey immediately after they finish the sixty-minute lesson or read my book, because the class involves hands-on activities which shock the student about what's really inside a cigarette. I invite you to dissect one cigarette while reading *14 & Out* and follow along as I take you on a quick journey through all of the major chemicals you find in one typical commercial cigarette. The ingredients include bleach, ammonia, glass wool and plastic. When you combine this cocktail of toxins and burn them, you create a vicious cycle that uses nicotine as the "aspirin" relief from the chemical hangover. *14 & Out* could be your way out of this vicious cycle.

Since 1997, I have built upon my master's degree in education from the University of Georgia to learn causes of and solutions to this insidious addiction. When I share the inside information I have researched and analyzed over the years from university research centers in the United Kingdom, Canada and in the U.S., smokers realize the depth of my research and my heartfelt commitment to their goal of quitting. I have interviewed doctors and nurses, received hundreds of testimonials from smokers who quit smoking by using *14 & Out*, and I have thoroughly researched every other cessation method available, from the patch to the gum, from electronic cigarettes to cold turkey. I've learned about the dangers of medications like Chantix and Zyban and their potential side effects.

I've interviewed hundreds of smokers about why they can't quit, including those who quit and went back to smoking. I've studied all the reasons people smoke, how they got started and why they can't stop. The FDA and the CDC may have limits and recommendations, but how much are they really helping or regulating the commercial cigarette industry?

I also figured out that the biggest part of the equation adding up to better health is eliminating dependence-enhancing or destructive chemicals from your food sources. I quit eating meat and became a vegetarian, but only after I learned what most U.S.-corporate-run farms and feed lots were doing to animals to "beef them up" and make more money. They give them hormones, and they abuse them by feeding them the wrong foods, like corn and genetically modified alfalfa, and the animals live in filthy, confined quarters, rarely if ever seeing sunlight. Then they give them antibiotics for their infections—lots of antibiotics. Then they slaughter them inhumanely, and the toxic meat is bleached and treated with ammonia, to make sure you don't get sick, at least initially, because if you got sick from it the same day, or a few days later, you could sue them or politicize it and ruin their name or brand. But when you eat it, you do get sick eventually, and you can end up with cancer of the prostate, or the bladder, or colon, or stomach and so on, all as a result of ingesting those hormones and chemicals. You can do the same thing with cigarettes. Learn to despise them for what has been done to trick you into becoming sick. Kill the urge, the desire, the "want of," and you cut the habit.

The success rates for smokers trying to quit are dismal. There are roughly forty-five million smokers in the United States alone, and half of them want to quit, yet only five percent who try to quit without help will succeed. The other ninety-five percent return to smoking in six months. That is a cold, hard fact. Scary commercials about cancer only motivate about four percent of people to quit smoking, according to the Centers for Disease Control and Prevention (CDC). The pills and the patch only help about ten percent to quit temporarily, if they're lucky, and electronic cigarettes, better known as "e-cigs" help even fewer, because most people remain addicted to nicotine, which is still highly toxic to cleansing organs like the liver and pancreas.

14 & Out is a natural way to escape smoking and what I call the "vicious cycle." No other program that I am aware of has the three main steps combined into one empowerment program. *14 & Out* has no gimmicks, no drugs, no hypnosis— just practical knowledge, behavior modification and nutrition.

With the highest success rate of any cessation program, this blows away the competition. No other book, video or class helps smokers quit and stay smoke free for life.

Every time someone quits smoking thanks to *14 & Out* I feel like my grandfather is smiling in Heaven, knowing I contributed something on this earth that saves thousands of people from what he went through. I tell you now, if you have the will, I have the way.

So, gather up your problems, your enemies, and your fears and flush them. We're going down to the basement of basics, to break everything down to its simplest form, so you can end the habit and get back to your healthy, happy life. When it's three in the morning and no one is awake but you, and you're looking in the mirror, wondering how everything came to this, you can smile and realize this is the first day of the rest of your phenomenal life without cigarettes! So get ready, because you are about to learn the secrets of the cigarette manufacturing process. You're about to learn the behaviors that have locked you into a potentially lethal habit. You are about to understand nutrition and exactly what your body needs to feel great so you don't crave another cigarette as long as you live.

If you would like to watch the preview/trailer for the 14 & Out sixty minute instructional video, link to it here:

http://premium.naturalnews.tv/14AndOut__TV.htm

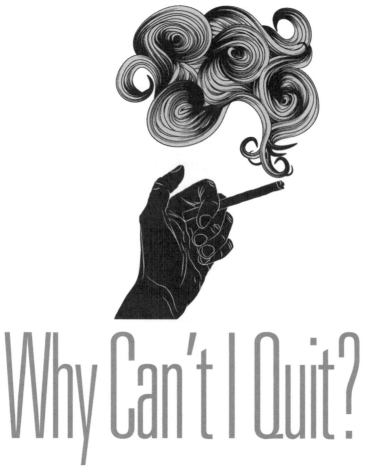

Why Can't I Quit?

Begin by asking yourself, "Why can't I quit?" Go ahead, say it out loud once. Why can't I quit? Any of these excuses sound familiar?

Smoking is just a break from work.

It's how you handle going back to work.

It helps you think about your problems.

It gets you out in the fresh air.

Your life is too stressful to quit smoking right now, maybe later.

Your friends smoke.

Your coworkers do it.

Your parents smoked, or your significant other got you started.

You are actually going through a breathing routine and a hand-to-mouth ritual that helps you relax.

The menthol ones help your chest and throat feel better.

It's how you wake up in the morning.

You need something to do.

It's a hand-to-mouth thing, kind of like a snack.

You like the ritual of it all.

It's legal!

You actually like it.

It looks cool.

It reduces stress!

You like sharing them.

It's just the perfect thing after a meal.

It's just a "social" thing.

You only smoke at bars and when you drink.

You only borrow or "bum" cigs, so it doesn't cost you anything! You just don't feel like quitting.

You can't quit.

You're going to quit soon, just not now.

You're going to quit one day because you're concerned about the effects on the people around you.

You can't deal with the stress of life without cigarettes.

You quit, and you are simply celebrating with this last one!

You have no idea why you smoke.

All the quitting methods failed you, so you just gave up.

You don't know how to quit.

No matter what the reason, you're about to learn. You see, most cessation programs fail because people have several different reasons why they smoke and why they can't quit, not just one or two. It's not just the nicotine! It's not just because nicotine relaxes you or gives you a little "pep." No other program in the world is unique in the way *14 & Out* recognizes that this habit and its cure are personal and specific to every individual. There are mental, emotional and physiological reasons people smoke, and there are mental, emotional and physiological reasons people can't quit, and that is exactly what we're addressing now. You can have all the motivation in the world to climb a mountain, but if you don't have a guide and the right tools, it can be quite difficult and full of surprises. Quitting smoking is like climbing a small mountain, so you need to get your "mind and body" in shape for this. Here we go!

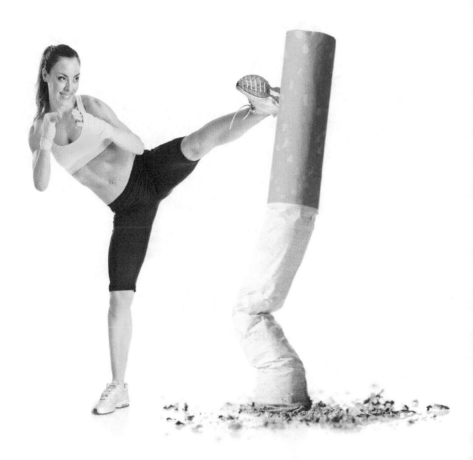

Part I
The Daily Guide

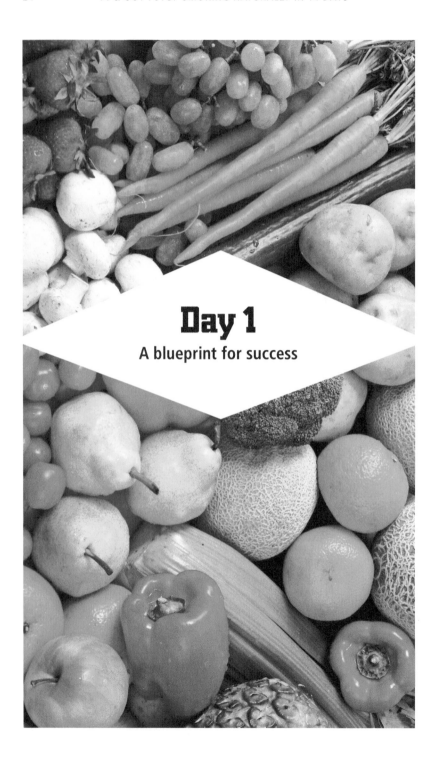

Day 1

A blueprint for success

Immediately go to a grocer, farmer's market or health food store and buy organic fruits and vegetables.

Make a salad at home and keep it simple with some or all of the following: kale, spinach, celery, cucumber, carrots, pickles, olives, onions and tomatoes. Buy organic dressing too. Make sure everything you buy is organic. You don't need to be eating pesticide while detoxifying from the four thousand chemicals that were in your cigarettes. If you don't want to eat salad every day or if it's too much roughage for your system, you can juice vegetables with a basic vegetable juicer, like the Jack LaLanne Juicer! They're cheap, maybe one hundred dollars or less, and they sell them at retail kitchen item shops or online! Then you begin a little exercise routine that you like. It should be easy, really easy at first so that it's fun. Stretch a little first so you're not sore the next day. That's key. Just go on a little jog or do some push-ups and crunches on your den floor, or jump rope outside or just go for a "fast" walk and burn a little energy. Get that heart rate up a little. Sweat a little. Keep it light. Fifteen minutes of cardio is a maximum starter. Smile as much as possible, as often as possible, even when things don't go your way.

The right supplements

Buy some recommended supplements. I'm not saying go break your wallet, or empty your purse or your bank account on supplements. I am saying that you have been wasting thirty-five dollars a week on cigarettes if you're a pack-a-day smoker and seventy dollars a week if you puff two packs a day. Spend that at first, then you can cut it in half after thirty days or so. It doesn't take a whole lot to supplement your body, but you need it, and you need it badly right now. Remember, every person's body is different, so there's no set guideline here, but here's a start: look for mucuna (dopabean) at a local vitamin shop or health food

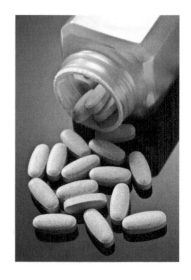

store. Ask the clerk. Sometimes it's listed as mucuna pruriens. It's very safe and natural. Also, you should shop for vitamin B complex with niacin. Again, ask questions about how much and when to take them. Your naturopath physician will also be a good guide here. That may take only a phone call. Then look at the amino acids, like tyrosine and glutamine. These will help repair and rebuild your muscles, muscle tissue, lung tissue that's damaged, throat and epithelial tissue and so on. Also look for some organic vitamin C supplements. You can't have too much vitamin C! Don't believe the myths. You can only have "expensive urine."

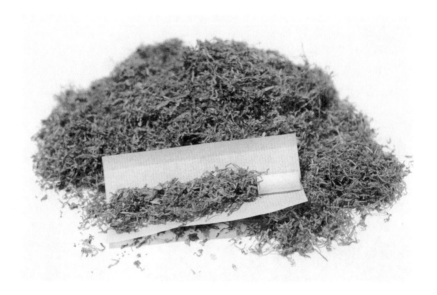

Organic tobacco

Buy organic tobacco at a smoke shop, tobacco shop or pipe shop near you. Some health food stores carry it. Also buy some rolling paper, preferably hemp or rice paper, or some other "unbleached" paper, so you're not smoking bleach. White paper is bleached. If you don't know how to "roll your own," just type those words in the YouTube search box and watch, or ask for help at the smoke shop. I'm sure you can learn quickly. It's well worth it. By making your own smokes you escape from the four thousand chemicals and the ammonia-enhanced nicotine. Only roll three a day, and only smoke three a day until the cravings decrease. Then thin that out to two, and then to one and then to NONE!

(http://www.naturalnews.com/034318_quit_smoking_method_organic_tobacco.html)

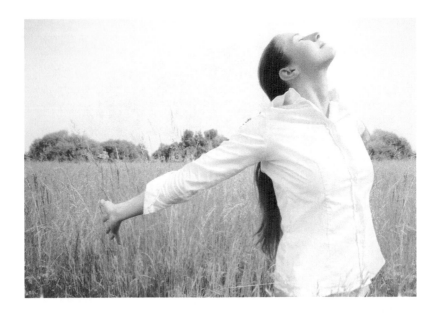

Breathe easy

Get outside for at least fifteen to twenty minutes, twice a day. If it's freezing cold or burning hot, make it ten minutes. You need the fresh air and the break. Do breathing exercises. <u>Pretend that you're holding a cigarette.</u> Put up two fingers next to each other, pretend to take a drag, inhale, hold for a second or two and then exhale. Do this over and over about ten to twelve times, or the same number of drags you would take if you were smoking. This will help break the ritual, the behavior habit you have of doing this motion hand to mouth, and you won't be ignoring your breathing pattern that makes you feel comfortable and relaxes you! <u>And now, you'll be breathing in fresh air instead of four thousand chemicals</u>!

Most people are familiar with hyperventilation, which is breathing in excess of what the body needs to eliminate carbon dioxide, but when most smokers do not have one "lit up," for some, they're breathing pattern is "hypoventilation," which is the opposite of hyperventilation, and occurs when breathing does not meet the body's needs, sometimes less than ten breaths per minute. This allows a build-up of carbon dioxide in the blood and decreases gas exchanges inside the lungs, and problems are compounded.

New research reveals the breathing pattern of smokers is the main part of the addiction. If you smoke a pack a day and take ten to twelve drags from each cigarette, that's two hundred and fifty times you breathe in and out in a specific way. Research surveys taken from hundreds of smokers who have kicked the habit show at least half realize, after going through the motions of breathing like when they have a cigarette, that the ritual is a major part of their addiction. <u>Be ready to start breathing as soon as you wake up.</u>

Coughing every morning is not natural. Why do smokers cough so much right when they get out of bed in the morning? And why does nothing come up? When you have a cold or congestion from allergies, sometimes you can cough up mucus and at least you can breathe or feel a little better. A person's breathing actually slows during sleep and for a smoker, that's when the tar moves in and settles on alveoli, which are the tiny air sacs in your lungs that contract and expand. So upon waking, a smoker feels like his or her chest is being compressed, as if he or she is choking just trying to get a full breath. That's why most smokers "cave" in the morning and light up, especially the menthol addicts. I've seen it with my best friends. I've lived with it. Breathe in the morning; flush your lungs.

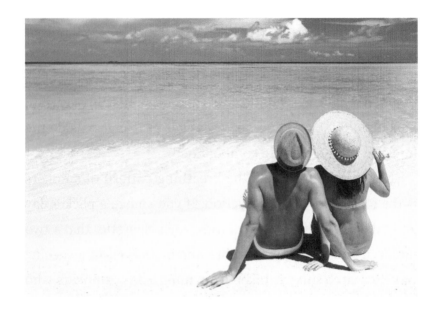

Speak humbly about quitting

Tell two special people you started this, but don't brag. Just mention it and see what they say. They will probably tell you about some way of quitting they heard about, and that's okay, because you have the best way, so just smile and listen. Then, think of a time, before you were a smoker, when you were healthy and having a good time. Visualize it: Maybe when you were on a vacation, a beautiful vacation somewhere like Hawaii, Mexico, the Bahamas, or just at a national park on a mountain, or at a lake or ocean. Maybe you were swimming in perfect blue water or walking through some gorgeous field, or maybe you were at the top of a mountain and could see for miles. <u>Keep this image in your head when you feel trapped inside, in an office, in an elevator, or in a long line somewhere.</u> Don't get antsy or impatient. Life is long. You are free. Think positively and use your mind's eye as your reliable friend!

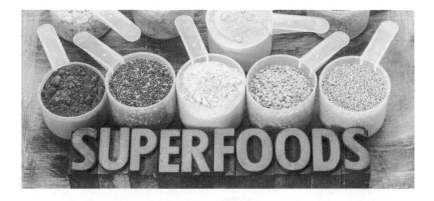

Superfoods

Staying alkalized will keep you from ever craving cigarettes again. Optimum health combined with despising cigarettes will free you for good. Understand and appreciate that Superfoods are core to your new food supplementing now and will help you gain pH balance in your body and blood. This is crucial for you now. Drink a mix of greens as a powder mix or a mix of red berries as a powder mix—they sell them at health food stores and vitamin shops. They sell them online at the Natural News store. But don't use milk to make shakes or smoothies, use rice milk or almond milk—they are much healthier! Make a shake before or after you exercise and take your supplements then, because the Superfood is a catapult for the nutrients in the supplements! Other powerful Superfoods include chlorella, spirulina, cacao, mangosteen, maca and coconut. Find out about all of these during your first six months as a nonsmoker! Also check out organic camu camu: http://store.naturalnews.com/Superfoods_c_4.html http://store.naturalnews.com/100-Organic-Camu-Camu-Powder-30oz_p_368.html

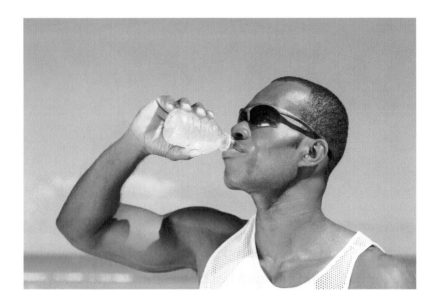

Spring water

Yes, spring water. You must drink spring water daily. Sip it when you have cravings. Sip it when you get a headache or need to digest a meal. Sip it to kill appetite. Trust me, with Superfoods and supplements you aren't going to put on a single pound of weight after you quit smoking. That's just a fallacy. People without a nutritional guide are the ones who put on weight. Plus, they're depressed and stressed, unlike you. You have a plan. You have this plan. Do not drink tap water. Filtered water is okay, but spring water is the key. It has dozens of minerals your body needs and wants, especially now.

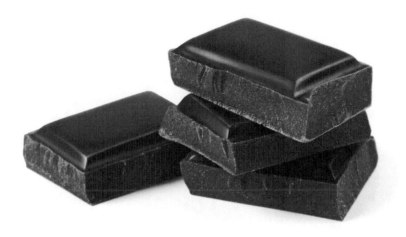

Organic chocolate

Of course, we are not talking here of the cheap candy bars you get at a convenience store or in line at the typical grocery stores. You need organic dark chocolate. It kills nicotine cravings and beats down depression. Break a bar into pieces and have little bites throughout the day or when you used to take cigarette breaks. This will help you a lot. This advice comes straight from ex-smokers who have taken my class and used this behavior modification skill. Put it to use and enjoy it all the while!

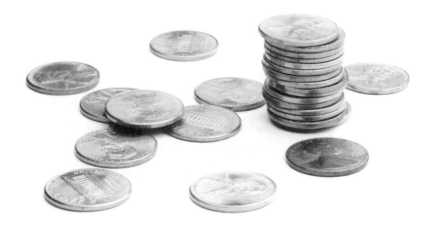

Don't be penny wise and pound foolish

Don't whine about the money for vitamins, supplements or Superfoods. <u>It's no more than a week's cost of cigarettes, plus you only need to restock about once a month, so that's about a fourth of what you spent on cigarettes—and this reverses all the damage!</u> Don't let anyone steer you away from this. Remember, people are like crabs in a barrel sometimes: If they see you escaping and they can't, they'll try to pull you back in. Stick to your guns. Stick to your convictions. Supplements are your way out.

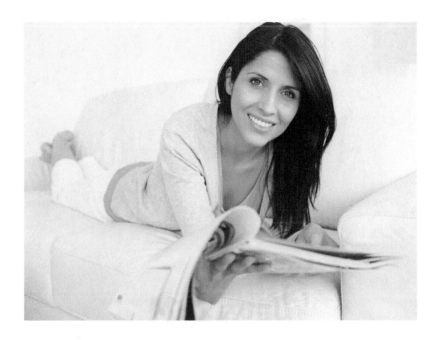

Educate yourself

Read health magazines and health articles online or at the library. Go to my favorite website in the world, NaturalNews.com, and check out a few articles each day. There are at least a dozen new ones every twenty-four hours, so you can keep your knowledge fresh and evolving. Also, you'll find an extensive Reference Guide at the end of this book.

http://www.naturalnews.com/index.html

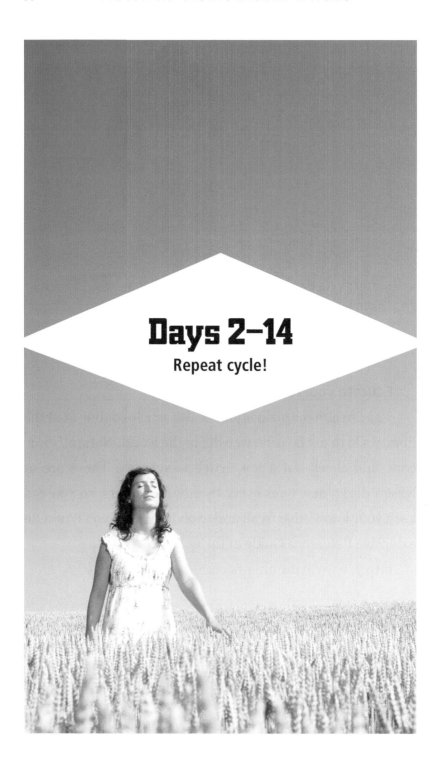

Days 2–14

Repeat cycle!

This may sound too easy, or too simple, but it's the perfect plan. <u>Repeat day one every day,</u> slowly weaning off of the organic tobacco and ramping up the nutrition.

You will notice improvement every day in energy, mood, vitality and overall well-being. Also, you must change your environment regularly. Don't forget, every time you "went out for a smoke" or changed where you smoked, you were changing your frame of mind and your scenery. <u>The idea is to break bad habits and replace them with healthy ones.</u> One way to do so is to physically remove yourself from those places where your bad habit, smoking, occurred. When you're trying to stop drinking it's probably best to avoid your favorite bar. It's the same idea. Choose new places to "go outside" for fresh air or to break from any monotony (boring routines). Turn this into a skill, and you'll feel the "release" of anxiety and become balanced, not needing or craving any kind of mood enhancer. Look to your organic snacks and supplements here.

Surviving the "crave" moments

Take work breaks without thinking about nicotine. How do you do that? Take "breathing ritual" breaks and snack on natural foods. Change your environment as often as you would when you smoked, especially at first. Mix it up with the supplements. Surprise your body here and there. Ask questions at your favorite vitamin shop and do research online using the websites I give you at the end of the book. Remember, your body can "get used" to repetition. It's your job to create

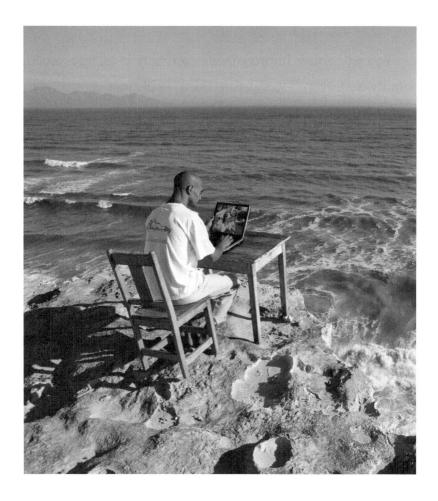

healthier repetition. You may vary your supplements, and ramp it up some (increase) at the beginning, and then back away a little as you go or just keep it steady. Again, everyone is different. You won't be doing it "wrong" if you just check out organic nutrients and ask questions at the vitamin shop and use your phone!

Call naturopathic physicians or even chiropractors and acupuncturists who often have a nutritional degree or some knowledge in this area. If you can afford it, check out these types of services. If not, just remember to surprise your body sometimes! See how your central nervous system feels! You're the best judge. Judge your temperament. Check your balance and your energy levels at different times of the day. Remember, herbs I mention such as mucuna are not a dire necessity right off the bat. Mucuna is great and it does help kill the nicotine cravings, but so will vitamin B complex with niacin and the organic chocolate. Don't think you can't start *14 & Out* the second you finish reading this book. If you choose to wait on the mucuna to arrive, or until you find it at the store, that's okay also. If you can't find mucuna at a store near you, go online to Puritan's Pride.com and buy it. Puritan's has low prices on many quality supplements, especially oil of oregano, which helps your body defend itself against viruses and allergies! Also check out colloidal silver and even just baking soda to help keep your body alkaline, instead of consuming foods and drinks that make the body/blood acidic, like soda, dairy, most meat and artificial sweeteners. That's covered in length coming up next.

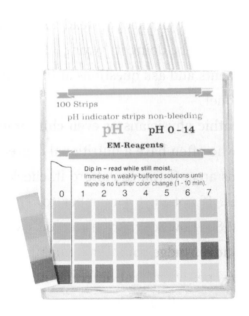

Test yourself

You can monitor your progress by measuring your own pH. Anyone can buy a pH testing kit (colored strips) and test their own pH daily for about a month for ten to twelve dollars. You simply wet a strip of paper with saliva and check the color against a key-coded strip you get with the little kit, and so you know instantly where you stand! An alkalized system will beat cigarettes, disease and cancer down and lead to perfect health. An acidic system depresses you, making you think you can't succeed, turning you negative, weak, sick, and craving habits you don't need. A person's pH can then be easily regulated within a few days, sometimes even hours, to be less acidic and more alkaline.

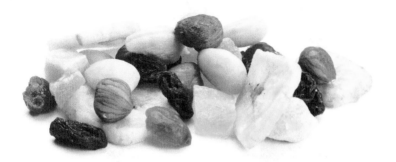

Hand-to-mouth tricks

Cut up some vegetables, like carrots or celery, and squirt some lime or lemon juice on them to help keep them fresh. Keep them with you, maybe in a sandwich baggie, at work or in your car or wherever you go. Also keep raw nuts with you, like trail mix with organic raisins or dark organic chocolate bits from your own unique mix. This will replace your hand-to-mouth ritual with something helpful to your body chemistry and energy. Beware of roasted nuts as they often make the body-blood more acidic.

The next vital step is to go all natural with the replacements for cigarettes. You see, sipping a drink all day, sucking on a sucker or nibbling on candy—these can all be hand-to-mouth habits, just like cigarettes. But you have the choice to go all natural and replace and replenish your system with nutrients while doing the hand-to-mouth motion. Raw mixed nuts, organic dark chocolate, spring water, dried organic fruits and berries, even taking supplements, will replace the hand-to-mouth motion and make you feel great.

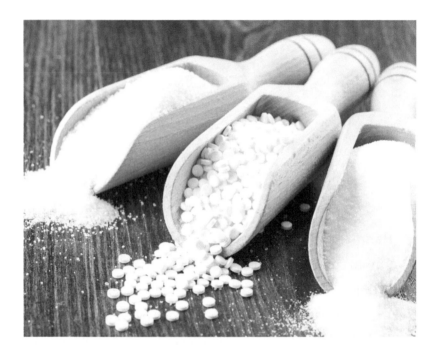

Avoid artificial sweeteners

Artificial sweeteners can wreck your plans for quitting cigarettes. Aspartame, sucralose, saccharine and sorbitol are the ingredients in Equal, Splenda, Sweet'N Low and Spoonful. They are synthetic and trick your body into craving more food and sugar. For some people these chemicals may damage the nervous system and digestive system! Avoid them at all costs. Some people may actually relapse from the chemicals and crave cigarettes again. Do not consume artificial sweeteners of any kind. Look for natural sugar substitutes like Stevia (not Truvia) and Xylitol.

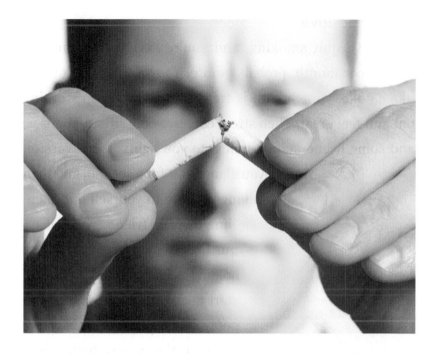

Stay strong

Even after quitting, a smoker's organs and central nervous system remain weakened from the chemicals for up to six months. This sickened state is what drives smokers back looking for relief, rather than the "nicotine addiction," which actually ends after three to five days. Other chemical imbalances can drive an ex-smoker to smoke also, like drinking alcohol often or abusively, or consuming aspartame or MSG (monosodium glutamate). Always remember this: It's the sickened chemical state of the central nervous system and the blood that drive smokers back to the well, not the nicotine. When you are stressed, your body wants organic food and organic beverages more than any other time!

Stay positive

You've quit smoking, and you're saving two hundred dollars per month, probably more. Your clothes don't smell like smoke, your breath is fresh and you've been working out and feel great. Then stress comes. Some situation arises, and some friend standing next to you lights up a cigarette. And so you glance at it for a second, and then you laugh a little to yourself and then, smiling at your friend, you put up your first two fingers, as if you're holding a cigarette, and pretend to start taking a drag. It may sound goofy, but it puts you in that state of mind—that you're better than that—better than the cancer sticks! You have a great purpose! So then take a nice deep breath, hold and exhale, and grab your water bottle or ask the waitress for a glass of water, knowing you're a nonsmoker who is never going back. It's all mental from there! Get ready for the ultimate shift of consciousness. When you stop flooding your system with toxins, and instead flood your system with nutrients and positivity, anything is possible.

If you like, you can turn to page 119 now and take the 20 question pre-quiz to see how much you know about your smoking habit. Then pick back up here and keep reading!

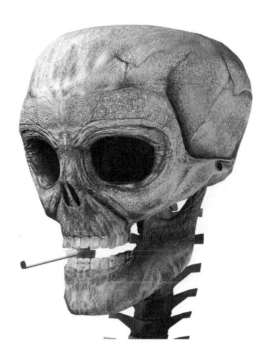

Thirty-three Things You Need to Know About Cigarettes & Smoking

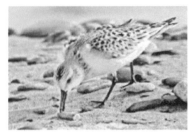

Animals can die from nicotine overdose.

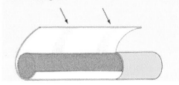

If a fire-safe cigarette is left unattended, the burning tobacco will reach one of these banded "speed bumps" and self-extinguish.

Fire-safe rungs are made of the same chemicals as carpet glue, so you're smoking even more chemicals with "safety" bumps.

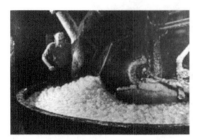

Commercial cigarette paper is bleached white, so you're actually smoking bleach.

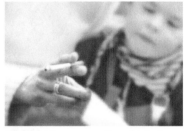

When kids see, smell and inhale secondhand smoke, damage is being done to more than just you, the smoker.

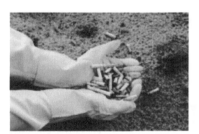

Cigarette filters (butts) can stick around the environment for fifteen years and pollute the earth.

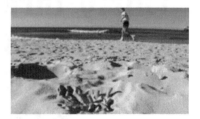

You always have the choice: Be part of the problem or be the solution. Stop polluting your insides and your "outsides."

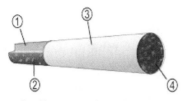

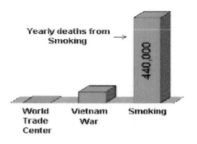

1. The filter is made with glass wool—fiberglass tears up your lung tissue.
2. Wrapping mats of cellulose acetate (photo film plastic) burn at seventeen hundred degrees.
3. Cigarette paper is bleached white, so you're smoking bleach.
4. Genetically modified tobacco contains pesticide—so you're smoking bug and weed killer.

Compared to other preventable tragedies, smoking blows them all away with horrific statistics. Don't be a statistic! Quit smoking.

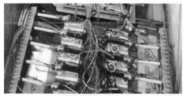

Commercial cigarettes are "efficient nicotine delivery devices" that fuel their own addiction to four thousand chemicals.

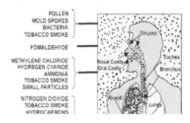

Your body is a machine, built to filter out toxins, but not four thousand per breath. Don't be a filter—quit naturally and get clean!

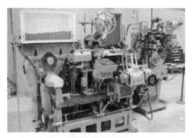

Tobacco companies use ammonia to freebase nicotine and make its potency up to thirty-five times as strong for your nicotine "hangover" relief system hook.

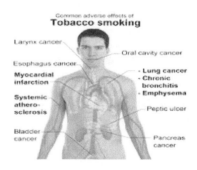

Are you racing toward cancer or away from it? You have complete control. Make your own decision with this life.

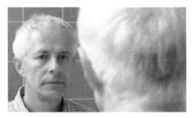

Face yourself. When all is said and done, just look yourself in the mirror and smile, knowing you are done smoking forever.

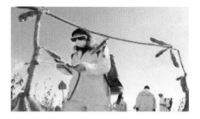

Ninety percent of tobacco is GMO, genetically modified to contain pesticide and is resistant or "immune" to plant poison, but YOU'RE NOT.

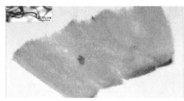

Cigarette papers are cross woven with plastic fibers to help them burn evenly so a cigarette won't blow out in heavy wind; so you're smoking plastic.

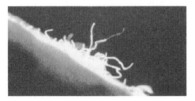

Just like asbestos, cigarette filters contain tiny "shards" of glass fibers that infect your lungs and tear the tissue apart over time.

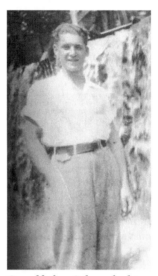

Grandfather Sol smoked two packs a day until he died of lung cancer. He is the reason I created the *14 & Out* program.

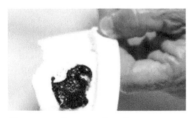

If you smoke a pack a day, you are putting two cups of tar in your lungs in just one year! It's time to detoxify.

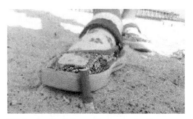

Kick the habit and never look back. Do it for your family, your children, yourself!

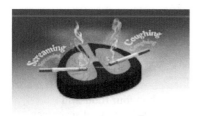

Your lungs are not an ashtray. Learn how to breathe free again, and free yourself from the nicotine prison.

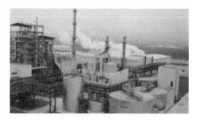

Your lungs are not a paper mill or some industrial waste complex. They are overloaded and burdened. End the habit.

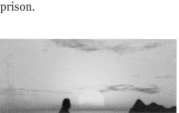

Meditation is a powerful force. Once you get your body clean, your mind will follow.

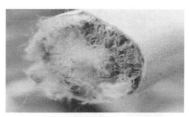

Ammonia, bleach, pesticide, plastic, fiberglass and tar equal death by choice. Choose life—quit smoking.

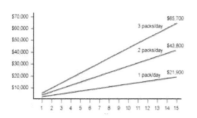

Do you smoke one, two or three packs a day? You could get a massage instead.

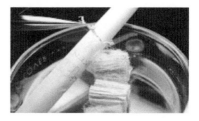

Dissect a cigarette and learn about what's really infecting your system, driving you to need another "fix."

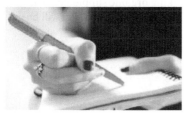

What's your New Year Resolution? Plan the work and then work the plan. Keep it simple with *14 & Out*!

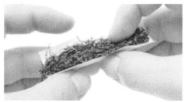

Roll your own organic tobacco during the fourteen days and remove the chemicals while weaning off nicotine!

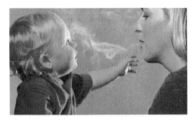

Most smokers underestimate the damage they are doing to others, including secondhand and thirdhand smoke (residue).

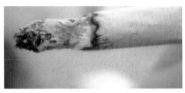

More than four thousand chemicals burning at seventeen hundred degrees during the inhale create the ultimate chemical "hangover." Your escape lives in nutrition and behavior modification.

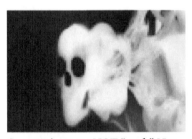

Cancer rings are NOT "cool." Non-smokers ARE cool. Become one and never look back.

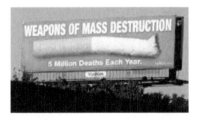

One Billion Deaths: Big Tobacco has been brainwashing people for seventy-five years, and cigarettes have killed more people than EVERY WAR put together.

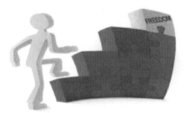

You don't have to re-invent the wheel. The steps to your freedom from cigarettes are set, just follow the "yellow brick road"—*14 & Out.*

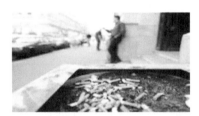

Your next "work break" will include eating Superfoods, taking organic supplements and breathing fresh air. You will be an ex-smoker for life!

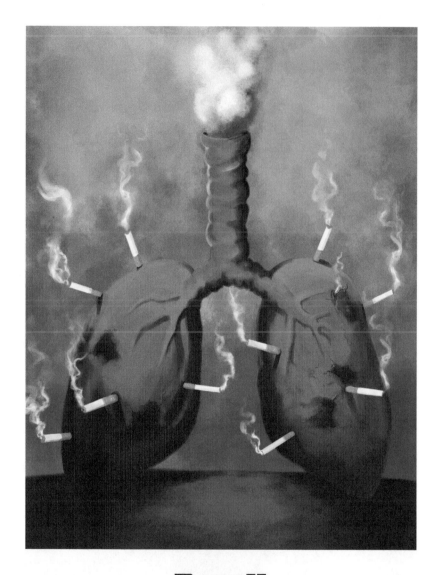

Part II
What Really Goes
Up In Smoke?

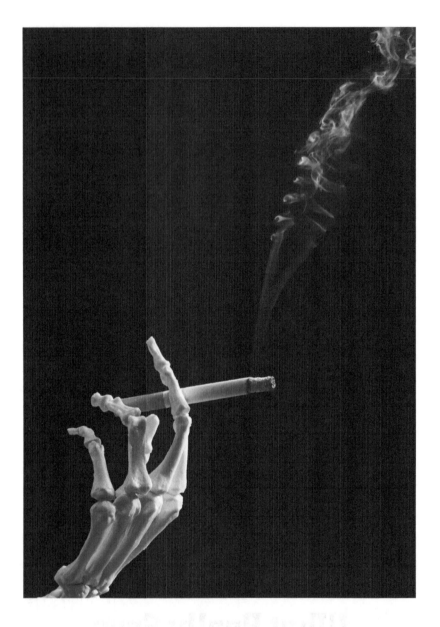

Now that you know how to quit the Big Tobacco addiction, it's time to discuss how you came to be a cigarette fiend in the first place. As you go through withdrawal, both behaviorally and physically, you will be more aware and better prepared to fight off the urges to light up again, if you understand what's happening in your brain and body. You'll know what to expect, and why.

Every inhaled puff of smoke contains free radicals which inflict damage on every system in the body, especially the digestive track and the intestines. Smoking increases the risk of Crohn's disease, gallstones, peptic ulcers and liver disease. The chemicals bond to the walls of healthy tissue in the esophagus, windpipe and stomach, disordering DNA and causing the cells to degrade. I'm sure you know lots of dangers of smoking, you've "heard them all before," but this is education about your vital organs, so bear with me for a minute. According to the American Diabetes Association, cigarette smoking has "demonstrable effects on blood sugar," making type two diabetes more likely. Smoking also ages the tissues of the pancreas, which creates defects in the digestive system. You cannot live without your pancreas.

Smoking impairs the lymphatic and immune systems, and can damage the soft tissue lining of the intestines. That's why colon cancer is prominent in smokers. Although the liver doesn't seem like part of the digestive system, it actually filters the nutrients and toxins from the blood in a process called first-pass metabolism. Smoking severely constricts this liver blood flow. After long-term use of nicotine, the body becomes dependent on it, recycling toxins back to the liver, and the result is constipation. The more you smoke, the worse it gets. The only solution is to get off nicotine and detoxify the liver, so e-cigarettes won't help.

So, what's causing all of this destruction? There's a lot more at work against you in that cancer stick then you might ever have imagined.

The chemicals in cigarettes have much more to do with the smoking addiction than nicotine. Let me say that again: The chemicals in cigarettes have much more to do with the smoking addiction than nicotine. Most cigarette smokers do not understand it's the chemicals in cigarettes that wreak havoc in their central nervous system, fueling the need for the short-lived relief nicotine brings. History proves that the premium brands contain more chemicals than others, and that is why they rule the market share and most of their "loyal smokers" will not even smoke the competition's brand because the "kick" or "taste" just isn't the same. What most fail to realize is that this desired kick and taste comes with a very steep price—that price being more pesticides, more ammonia and a richer toxic cocktail that does damage to the lungs and nervous system in the short term.

If all cigarette manufacturers today faced strict and thorough inspections and regulations, and had no choice but to eliminate all of the chemicals, the number of cancer cases would be reduced immensely and the ability to stop smoking without help would be reasonable again.

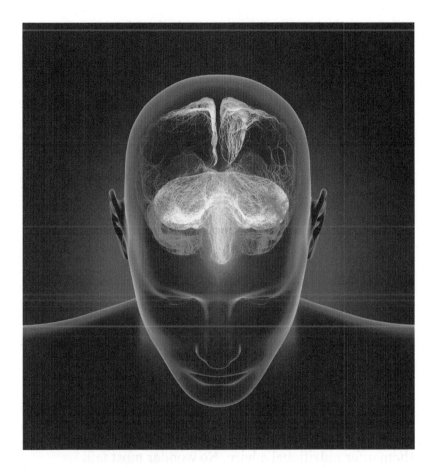

Nicotine and dopamine

Stimulants produce short-lived euphoria, but then it goes away and needs more synthetic stimulation, hence, the chemical addiction and the vicious cycle. With repeated use, stimulants can disrupt the functioning of the brain's dopamine system, dampening users' ability to feel any pleasure at all. Users may try to compensate by taking more and more of the drug to experience the same pleasure. Dopamine functions in your brain to help you deal with stress, anxiety and relaxation, and should be naturally occurring, not chemically induced. Your body could actually stop creating natural reactions that help you relax or motivate you to deal with stress. You are getting "false confidence" using nicotine.

Nicotine gum delivers between two and four milligrams per piece. It fails as a way to break the habit because this is nothing close to the amount received from smoking an ammonia-treated "cig." The nicotine patches deliver less than one mg. (between .5 and .9 mg) each hour, and that's on a slow, fairly constant release into the blood. Again, that's nothing like the nicotine vapors in a commercial cigarette, which reach the heart and brain within three seconds. Like we covered a little earlier, medications like Chantix and Zyban do not contain nicotine at all, but block the brain's receptors to it, creating a very dangerous "wall," which can also disrupt dopamine and serotonin from reaching proper regions in the brain. This is exactly why suicide is a side effect of these two prescription medications. These programs are nothing like smoking, and do not wean you off the nicotine. Plus, none of them offer nutritional advice. No wonder most fail.

Visualize the war that's going on inside your brain; nicotine versus dopamine. Natural fight or flight reactions are now becoming nervous disorders. Organic feelings and emotions about life in general become exaggerated problems which seem insurmountable at times. After long-term use of high-potency cigarettes, a person can permanently cripple the dopamine system and ruin the ability to feel pleasure at all without smoking a cigarette. Understanding and addressing the chemistry of it all is the cure. Dopamine functions in your brain to help you deal with stress, anxiety and relaxation, and should occur naturally, instead of being chemically induced.

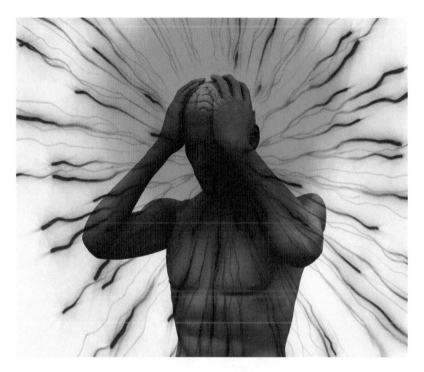

This is what cigarette manufacturers realized fifty years ago, and this is the hook that keeps smokers addicted and pulls them "back in" when they quit.

Medications don't contain nicotine at all, but block the brain's receptors to it, which is very dangerous and creates side effects. Because the medications also block your dopamine, this causes some smokers to commit suicide. Just one juiced up commercial cigarette delivers between fifty and one hundred milligrams of nicotine potency. Organic tobacco in self-rolled cigarettes contains only ten to twelve milligrams of nicotine. So you see, understanding the war between nicotine and dopamine helps smokers quit!

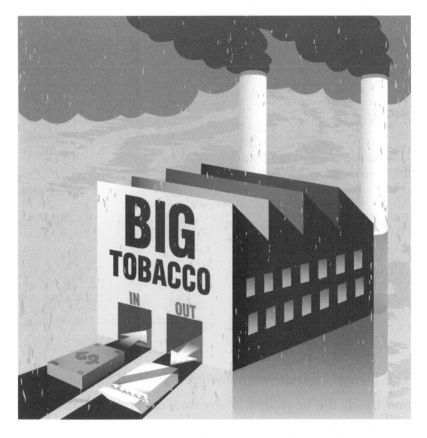

Ammonia and the dark history of "Big Tobacco"

Nearly all cigarette manufacturers use ammonia to boost the impact of nicotine so it is more quickly absorbed by the lungs. This process of converting the nicotine from an acid form to a base form is known as "freebasing" and leads to a more intensely addictive nicotine experience for seasoned smokers and a much faster road to addiction for a new smoker. In this chemically altered form, nicotine deposits directly on the lung tissue and is immediately distributed throughout the body. This experimentation started in the 1970s, when Marlboro and Kool figured out that low-tar cigarettes had lower nicotine levels which diminished the smoker's overall "experience," and so scientists figured out that ammonia would free up nicotine molecules so they would vaporize more easily into a gas and heighten the addictive quality of the more popular lower-tar cigarettes by increasing the "nic-fit" sensation by as much as one hundred times.

Marlboro and Kool enjoyed increased market shares and profit margins so much greater than most other brands, that they almost put the competition out of business.

In 1965, scientists at R.J. Reynolds were trying to find out why Winston was losing ground to Philip Morris's Marlboro brand, and in their research discovered that Marlboro contained ammonia compounds. In the 1970s, Reynolds started adding ammonia and "slowly but surely, everyone fell in line." By 1990, documents showed that tobacco companies were using more than ten million pounds of ammonia compounds each year. Researchers at Oregon Health and Science University used a laboratory smoking device to collect and analyze smoke from eleven brands of cigarettes. The study measured the first three puffs of smoke from each cigarette. http://*14andout*.blogspot.com/2013/08/the-secret-of-marlboros-success.html

The dosage or "potency" of one commercial cigarette is actually more than one hundred milligrams of nicotine, but that potency doesn't register on nicotine level testers because cigarette manufacturers use ammonia to supercharge nicotine to hit your brain in less than three seconds. Brands that deliver the "nic hit" (nicotine burst) the quickest and strongest often have the best sales and brand loyalty. They used to call the nicotine-treated tobacco that "roasty, toasty

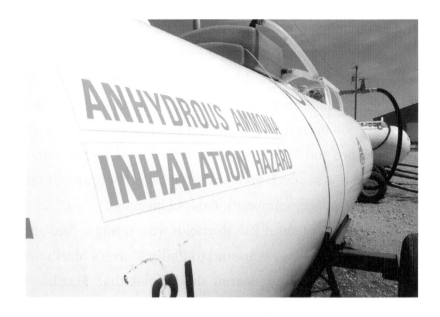

flavor," until they got caught.

http://www.prwatch.org/spin/2008/06/7479/secret-marlboros-success-freebase-nicotine

Do you remember Jolt Cola? It was that cola that had massive amounts of caffeine but not quite as much as today's Red Bull or Monster! People actually overdose from energy drinks like Monster and it's well-documented. What if there was a beer or wine that hit the shelves that had a third more alcohol content than typical, but it didn't say anything on the label about it? What if you chugged three or four, thinking it was pretty much all the same, and you wrecked because of it, or ended up in the emergency room? Could you imagine the car wrecks, the DUI's, the overdoses and the court cases that would ensue because of it?

Most of the premium brands of cigarettes have more nicotine potency than you think, and the manufacturers don't have to label them as such. That's a part of the problem with tobacco regulation and FDA labeling. To find out exactly what is crippling your central nervous system and your immune system, one has to literally dissect cigarettes, which is what I've done for you, and this is a big part of what I am communicating to you now. In the *14 & Out* live class, my students (clients) cut open a cigarette and the filter, and we bring out magnifying lenses, and they have to look at the ingredients up close and smell the toxic chemicals. This puts a shock in your soul and your eyes and your nose and your brain. Perspectives change when smokers realize what they're really inhaling. They see the glass fibers in the filter and mix them with tar (I use toothpaste or black caulking for effect). You get your fingers in the mess that your lungs are dealing with all the time.

When smokers smell the sample of the ammonia, the bleach, and most of all, the pesticide that I bring to class, they are better motivated to quit. If you have those cleaning chemicals around the house, when you take a break from reading this, go take a little sniff of a few, and you will understand these topics a little better. Then imagine inhaling those vapors all day, every day. You'll want to quit for good.

Think about this for a second—why don't cigarettes go out in heavy wind? You can hold your cigarette out the car window while driving down the road and it won't go out. Why? You think it's just tobacco and regular rolling paper? Try rolling your own and see what happens.

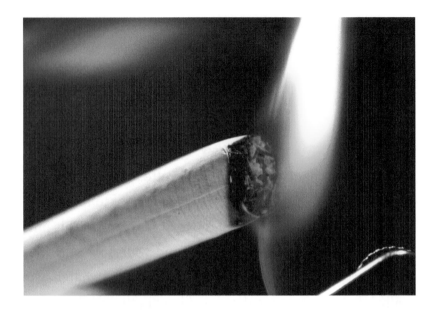

Plastic and carpet glue

That's correct; wrapping mats are cross woven with cellulose acetate to burn hot and evenly. Ever been touched and burned by the lit end of a cigarette? I have. I still have the scar on top of my right hand, thirty-five years later. The tip of the cigarette burns at about seventeen hundred degrees Fahrenheit during the inhale and over one thousand degrees when idle between drags. You think that's just paper and tobacco burning?! Think again. You're burning cellulose acetate—a plastic used in photo film!

That's why there are so many house fires started from cigarettes, even the "fire-safe" ones, which are loaded with extra "carpet glue" rings. You are burning over 4,000 chemicals, including ammonia and pesticide. That means you are smoking bug and worm killer with every cigarette, every drag. Take a cigarette and cut it in half long ways, so you cut the stem that holds the tobacco and the little spongy filter. Spread everything out with your fingers, and if you have a magnifying glass, grab it. Ever wonder why cigarettes burn so evenly, from start to finish? They never trail up one side. Are they wrapped in simple paper, or is there more to it than that? Is something flammable weaved carefully into the paper that wraps the tobacco? You bet your last five bucks there is!

Think of how big of a joke "fire-safe cigarettes" are now! The safety "rings" or toxic "rungs" are made of an ethylene- vinyl-acetate-copolymer-emulsion-based adhesive (carpet glue), which causes severe irritation of mucous membranes and the upper respiratory tract. Symptoms of this damage include a severe burning sensation, laryngitis, shortness of breath, headaches, nausea and vomiting!

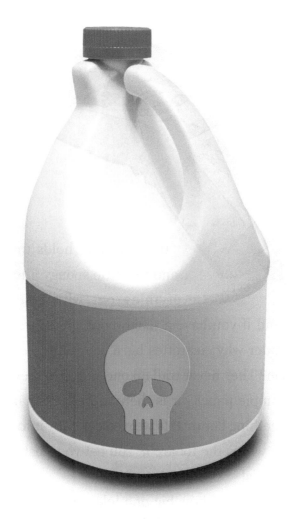

Bleach

Trees are not white, they're brown, but most cigarettes are white. They're bleached. Since the paper has been dyed white with bleach, that means you're smoking bleach. Yes, it does. You're burning it and breathing it in, over and over again, and that's just the beginning. Did you know that when you mix ammonia with bleach and burn it, it becomes a form of lethal mustard gas. Never try it at home—you could choke to death; just leave that "modern science" laboratory work up to the professionals who are making cigarettes. What happens when you burn pesticides, insecticides and weed killers like Roundup? That's what they spray in huge doses on the tobacco plants to keep away bugs and weeds! You better believe it's a cocktail of poisons. And now corporations bio-engineer, meaning they inter-splice Roundup pesticide with seedlings in order to grow plants (corn, soy, tobacco, etc.) that are actually composed of weed killer—that way the plants are immune to the chemicals, no matter how much they use. It's called GMO, genetically modified organisms.

What about us humans? Research shows these companies use up to fifteen times more pesticide on genetically modified vegetation (GMO) and the plants live through it. The EPA has also raised the tolerance level of pesticides for human consumption. They obviously are not out to protect us.

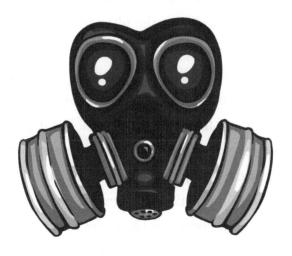

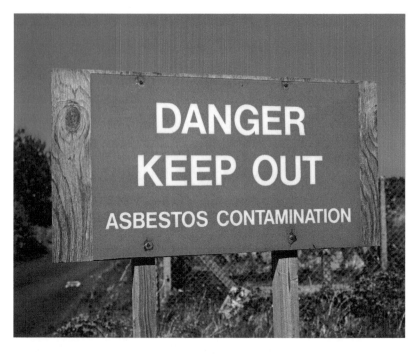

Asbestos

Why does it take up to fifteen years for a cigarette filter to disintegrate? If the cigarette filter was just cotton and paper, and I threw it in the yard, it would be gone after a couple of rainstorms. What also keeps the filter from getting hot? Is it cotton or some form of a sponge? You can smoke it down to the nub, and your fingers won't even get warm. How is it insulated? Could it be some kind of glass fibers, maybe some form of glass wool or fiberglass insulation, like in your attic?

Glass wool, fiberglass, fibrous glass and glass fibers are all names for the same thing: thin, needle-shaped rods of glass, which nature does not make, but humans do. If you've ever come in contact with fiberglass, like in your attic, you already know what it can do to your skin. The tiny fibers of glass from insulation wool can irritate your skin and eyes.

If you experience too much contact with fiberglass, it can cause what's called irritant contact dermatitis, or inflammation of the skin. Breathing in glass fibers can also increase the difficulty of breathing. Ever wake up in the morning and have a coughing fit you can't seem to escape from? There's also a plastic called cellulose acetate in the filter. Cellulose acetate is what's used to make photo film. Smoking plastic affects your (CNS) central nervous system, leading you to crave relief from the damage. Fiberglass became popular in the United States as asbestos was phased out. Asbestos, unlike fiberglass, is a naturally occurring silicate material found in rocks. Its known use goes back to the ancient Greeks, who admired it for its ability to withstand very high temperatures. Indeed, asbestos isn't just resistant to heat. It also doesn't evaporate in the air, dissolve in water or react with most chemicals. Think now of why cigarette filters aren't biodegradable. When breathed in, asbestos and fiberglass fibers go deep into the lungs, where they stay for long periods of time. During that time, the fibers irritate the lungs and any other part of the body they may travel to, disrupting cell division by interfering with chromosome distribution and changing important genetic material.

Asbestos is classified as a known human carcinogen by state, federal and international agencies, and new uses of the material were banned in 1989 by the Environmental Protection Agency. Still, we frequently see asbestos-related problems, from the evacuation of poorly constructed school buildings to debris created from Hurricane Katrina in New Orleans in 2005. While asbestos is a natural material and fiberglass is man-made, the two materials are often compared because they're both fibrous. Fiberglass also has the heat-resistant qualities that made asbestos so desirable for insulation. When it's mid-summer, one hundred degrees outside and the sun is beating down on your roof but you're sitting in sixty-eight degrees of air conditioning inside, like a hotel room, it's because the insulation acts as a buffer to the heat.

Now, think of why cigarette filters don't get hot! You can smoke a cigarette right down to the filter, and your fingertips don't even get warm! The manufacturers did what was convenient for more sales, knowing good and well it kills you. Here's the kicker: Fiberglass can be just as dangerous as asbestos—and it's sometimes referred to as the "asbestos of the 20th century."

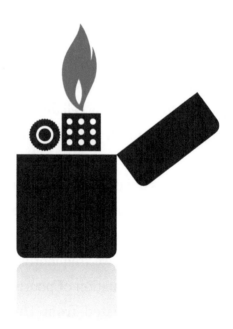

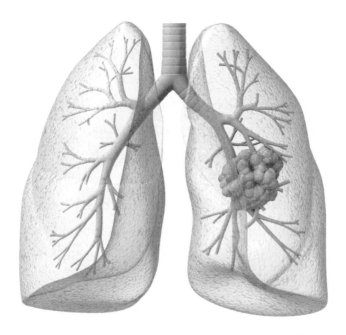

What's going on in your lungs?

A study in 1970 on rats stated that "fibrous glass of small diameter is a potent carcinogen." Studies have continued to show that fibers of this size not only cause cancer in laboratory animals, but also cause changes in the activity and chemical composition of cells, leading to changes in the genetic structure and in the cellular immune system. So we have to ask: How can this not apply to mankind?

When I first designed *14 & Out* and taught classes at the local libraries, people kept asking me for proof that cigarette filters contain fiberglass or "glass wool," so instead of just dissecting the filters in class and comparing them to the fiberglass right in front of the students, I decided to dig deeper. I conducted several interviews with professionals in the medical field, and they have seen the proof in lung X-rays of their patients. They told me about it, and I documented everything. This confirmed all of my research and gave me even more inspiration to share. A specific type of lung cancer many smokers develop comes from *tiny tears* in their lung tissue caused by microscopic glass fibers, also known as glass wool, found in many conventional cigarette filters. These rips in the epithelial (soft) tissue fuel the development of tumors and cancerous cells due to the constant overload of toxins, namely pesticides, nicotine and ammonia, contained in commercial cigarette smoke. This rips apart the tissue and helps the chemicals get into your lungs and do more damage.

This is important, so let me explain again. The filters of typical commercial cigarettes contain microscopic, needle-shaped shards of glass wool which escape into the mouth and throat and then lodge with tobacco tar in the lung tissue, surrounding the alveoli (tiny air sacs) and leading to **COPD** (chronic obstructive pulmonary disease), emphysema and eventually lung cancer.

One killer linked to asbestos is mesothelioma, a deadly cancer that develops in the protective lining of the lungs, abdomen and/or the cavity around the heart, and it is most commonly associated with asbestos poisoning. Research reveals that more than ten percent of those cases are now associated with cigarette smokers with no history of exposure to asbestos ... coincidence?

There are no toxicological examinations by the tobacco industry that I can find assessing the human health risks from inhaling and ingesting these synthetic microparticles released from conventional cigarettes.

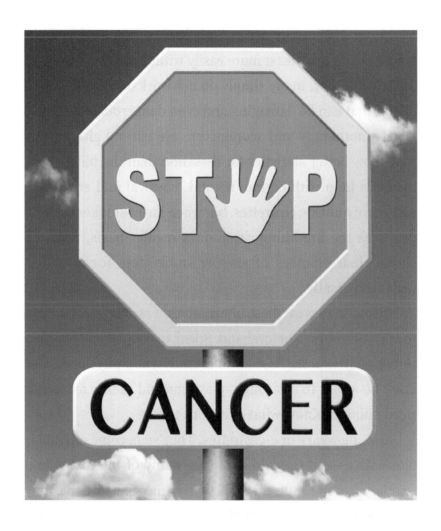

Part III
Dangerous Alternatives

There are lots of drugs and devices invented to help smokers quit or at least more easily withdraw from smoking. As I said earlier, many simply do not work or they have side effects that can be damaging and even dangerous.

Hypnotherapy and acupuncture are natural alternatives that show better statistics for cessation than the pills. These methods help with certain mental, physical and emotional aspects of quitting cigarettes, but when an ex-smoker actually practices the breathing ritual on a regular basis, research shows their chances of staying smoke-free for good are increased greatly.

If you do choose these alternatives, I strongly advise you to educate yourself beforehand. Speak to trained and licensed nutritional experts first and certainly your physician. But don't be afraid to ask tough questions and seek a second or third opinion. Know what questions to ask.

Also, be weary of e-cigarettes. They've become a popular alternative—and they do eliminate many of the toxins in a regular cigarette. But, they still deliver nicotine into the body and may have some potential dangers of their own. Plus, they receive even less government oversight than tobacco-based products because they are considered a "delivery system," not a drug.

Here is a brief look at some of what I call the *dangerous alternatives* to quitting the right way—the safe way—the *14 & Out* way.

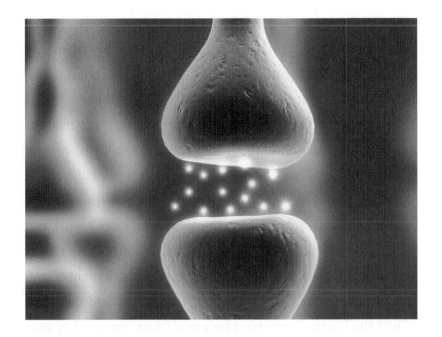

Chantix

Smoking cessation pills simply make anxiety and depression worse. Chantix blocks nicotine receptor sites in the brain in order to reduce nicotine cravings, but in that process, naturally occurring dopamine and serotonin are blocked, creating dangerous and nearly intolerable side effects.

When a human being experiences a stressful or exciting event, natural hormones create neural reactions in the brain's central processing area called synapses, which involve neurons firing electrical charges that stimulate behavior and mood elevations. Chantix can **block these natural reactions** from doing their job, sometimes preventing the person from coping with anxiety, depression and frustration. Chantix sometimes can disable the natural "fight or flight" reaction, which in turn can, for some people, make even small problems seem insurmountable, leading to feelings of intense anxiety and thoughts of suicide. Please understand how tragic this is, even for people who are fairly stable and sane! Even the petty problems and stress from simple frustrations can become overwhelming in an instant. Some little problem will haunt you all day as if it's a major issue you can't solve. Your brain simply cannot work it out during the day and the stress builds up subconsciously. Your mind can't work out your basic problems or get past miniscule obstacles. This is why sleeplessness and nightmares, very strange nightmares, are a side effect of these lab-concocted, synthetic drugs. This is just the beginning of your new problems, and so they may get you off cigarettes, maybe, but then you're in need of some antidepressants or "lobotomizing" drugs for life.

Chantix, chemically known as varenicline, has side effects which include agitation, depression and onset of psychiatric illness such as psychosis, mania, bipolar disorder, schizophrenia and hallucinations.

Chantix may lead to the recurrence of old psychiatric illness. Some patients have attempted or committed suicide. The Institute for Safe Medication Practices reported that Chantix accounted for more "serious drug adverse events" in the United States than any other drug in 2008. Can you imagine? The FDA issued alerts about some of these serious adverse side effects. At one point, the Chantix label was updated to mention reports of depression, agitation, changes in behavior and suicide. Still considering taking Chantix? Here's the list of side effects directly from the website:

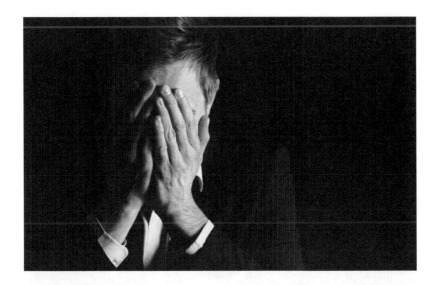

"Some people have had changes in behavior, hostility, agitation, depressed mood, suicidal thoughts or actions while using CHANTIX to help them quit smoking. Some people had these symptoms when they began taking CHANTIX, and others developed them after several weeks of treatment or after stopping CHANTIX. If you, your family, or caregiver notice agitation, hostility, depression, or changes in behavior, thinking, or mood that are not typical for you, or you develop suicidal thoughts or actions, anxiety, panic, aggression, anger, mania, abnormal sensations, hallucinations, paranoia, or confusion, stop taking CHANTIX and call your doctor right away. Also tell your doctor about any history of depression or other mental health problems before taking CHANTIX, as these symptoms may worsen while taking CHANTIX."

Are you kidding me? How can doctors legally prescribe this and in good faith? How does the FDA and the CDC allow these horror drugs on the market?

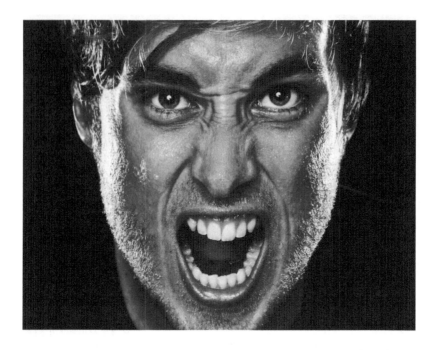

Zyban

Zyban, chemically known as bupropion, is actually an antidepressant. The most common side effects of Zyban are agitation, dry mouth, insomnia, headache, nausea, constipation and tremor. What person in their right mind needs to experience tremors while they are trying to quit cigarettes? Some patients may experience weight loss. Seizures also occur, especially at higher doses. Research published in 2010 in the *American Journal of Obstetrics and Gynecology* suggested that women who take Zyban during early pregnancy run a greater risk for having a baby born with a heart birth defect. That's just crazy. You quit smoking to help the baby have good cells and good health and now the child has a birth defect. Not a good plan, if you ask me.

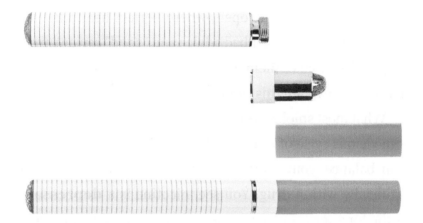

E-cigs (electronic cigarettes)

You need to escape the "nicotine prison" all together, and go from "cigs" to "no cigs," not from cigs to e-cigs. You see, it's tough to criticize electronic cigarettes completely because some of those who use them can brag that they have eliminated most of the toxic chemicals found in commercial cigarettes, and that they're saving money and may have cut back on how often they smoke. About one out of every three e-cig "fans" will tell you they quit smoking entirely thanks to e-cigs, and that's great, but what happened to the other two-thirds?

It is true that e-cigs have a better success rate for helping smokers quit than the nicotine patch, the gum, the medications (Chantix and Zyban) and hypnotherapy combined, according to the *American Journal of Preventive Medicine*. But the ultimate irony is that e-cigs were never meant to be marketed as a quit-smoking aid, according to the inventors from Hong Kong. People just want a way out, and e-cigs shine a little bit of light at the end of that tunnel. But what if, instead of shining a little "light at the end of the tunnel," we get you free, out into the great wide open, where perfect health is your new frontier? People get bad advice and "good" reviews from e-cigs, and it makes them think nicotine is okay to smoke. It's not. Let me explain this thoroughly.

What most smokers don't realize is that nicotine creates its own vicious cycle of ***need and feed***. This is still controlling your balance, your central nervous system and your moods artificially with a drug. You see, nicotine is a **depressant** in the long term but serves as a short-term stimulant, so it actually relieves the smoker of the very feeling it created, which has quickly worn off from the last smoking session, usually thirty to forty minutes earlier. In other words, a few nicotine drags are like taking aspirin for an alcohol hangover, over and over, and smokers engage in this "hangover relief system" about once an hour, some twice (two packs a day). It's a hook and an evil drug from which the body wants to escape. There are currently no regulations whatsoever of the ingredients in e-cigs and no age restrictions for purchasing them either. This "hot" new product is marketed to children, teens and adults, and is sold in shopping malls at kiosks and on hundreds of websites.

Nicotine doses in e-cigs have an enormous range, from a mild five milligrams, on up to sixty milligrams. Botched jobs by amateur manufacturers can end up delivering over three hundred milligrams, which is a possible lethal dose, especially for a child or teenager who has either low or no tolerance for it. That's three times the nicotine of your average commercial cigarette today! Imagine putting three cigarettes together and smoking all three at once. How would you feel? Like a nervous wreck. Also, the nicotine levels on the cartridges are often wrong, and research reveals that many of the e-cigs that claim they are nicotine-free are not. Do not believe all the hype. What has been made to look "cool" in magazines and advertisements is a trick and just another health disaster. Trust me on this.

E-cigs are very tough for the FDA to regulate, mainly because they are not actually tobacco products but simply nicotine delivery devices. I've read plenty of reviews and blog comments about e-cigs. People brag and say it helped them get off all those chemicals in cigarettes, or maybe that they went to e-cigs and then they quit smoking shortly after that. More power to you, but for most people, nicotine continuance is just sugar-coating the problem. The benefits and "safety" of e-cigs are *quite misleading*. Here's what I found. There are twenty varieties of e-cigs that contain **nitrosamines,** the same carcinogen found in real cigarettes, and most e-juice (nicotine juice) cartridges contain diethylene glycol, the highly toxic poison found in antifreeze, which causes leukemia.

Many e-cigs which claim to have no nicotine will contain some, and many of the levels of nicotine disclosed on the packages are completely wrong, so it's kind of a guessing game as to how much "drug" you're getting and which manufacturers actually know what they're doing when they "load them up." Today in America, e-cig devices are available in over three thousand retail outlets and all over the Internet. They cost anywhere between forty-five and seventy-five dollars, and sales have skyrocketed in the past year, exceeding one hundred million.

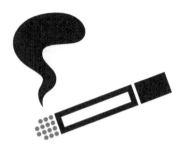

Common questions about smoking alternatives

1. Are e-cigs legal all over the world? Australia and Canada have banned e-cigs, classifying them as a tobacco product. Though the e-cig does not contain tobacco, those governments won't make the exception. As far as the U.S. is concerned, national border security is confiscating e-cigs, but there is no law banning their use yet. However, since they're quickly depleting Big Tobacco's profits, the FDA will likely step in very soon!

2. What really happened to the guy in Florida whose e-cig blew up in his face? Tom Holloway of Niceville, Florida, is still alive, but is missing half his tongue, all of his front teeth and has permanent burn scars on his face. This is a true story: http://www.naturalnews.com/035026_e-cigarettes_ explode_teeth.html

3. What are the side effects of nicotine? Nicotine by itself causes an increased heart rate, heightened blood pressure, narrowing of blood vessels (leads to heart attacks

and strokes), gastrointestinal problems, depression, mood swings, sleep disturbances, headaches, loss of your sex drive, insulin resistance and vision problems.

4. Just how addicting is nicotine, really? Nicotine is one of the most addictive drugs in the world, running a close third behind heroin and cocaine. The physical addiction is actually broken in three to four days, but the cravings for the feelings that nicotine brings can take weeks, months or even years to stop without the proper nutritional and herbal replacement and replenishment supplements. Therefore, many smoking alternatives, like e-cigs, are just a hook into another addiction or unhealthy habit.

5. How are the stop smoking pills like Chantix and Zyban dangerous? These pharmaceutical toxins not only block nicotine receptors in the brain but also block naturally occurring dopamine, so the patient suffers from heightened depression and anxiety, which fuels feelings of suicide and can even lead the patient to commit suicide.

6. How is *14 & Out* different from all other quit-smoking programs? *14 & Out* addresses the chemical addiction, behavioral patterns and rituals, and nutritional guidance so desperately needed to quit smoking for good. If you feel incarcerated by the nicotine addiction, you now have the key to free yourself from your nicotine cell.

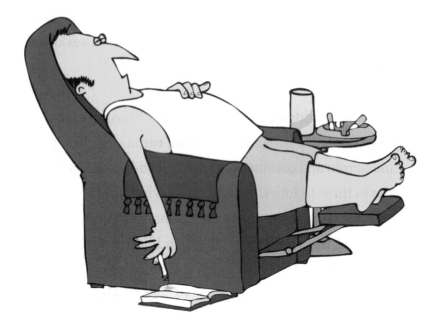

Fire-safe smokes

There has been some buzz about the creation of "fire-safe" cigarettes for those who won't quit but want to feel less threatened. To me, this technology is just another reason provided to keep smoking—and may even make your quit tougher. The real rationale for the creation of fire-safe cigarettes wasn't so much for consumer protection, but was meant more for the manufacturers' defense against lawsuits if and when a smoker accidentally burns their house down. Prior to the introduction of the fire-safe cigarette (FSC), commercially rolled cigarettes (unlike cigars) would burn all the way down to the filter if left unattended. Despite claims that they are safer, however, a fire-safe cigarette still burns for over a minute between safety rings, also known as "speed bumps," and so the number of fires caused by unguarded lit cigarettes has barely been reduced. That's the bad news.

Unfortunately, there is no good news. The other bad news is that the "safety rings" are made of an ethylene-vinyl-acetate-copolymer-emulsion-based adhesive (carpet glue), which causes severe irritation of mucous membranes and the upper respiratory tract. Symptoms of this damage include a severe burning sensation, laryngitis, shortness of breath, headaches, nausea and vomiting. In other words, the speed bumps are not only useless, but they are compounding problems for smokers.

Many smokers know the risks involved in falling asleep with a lit cigarette, but cigarette manufacturers and corporations needed some added insurance against lawsuits, so they created the fire-safe cigarette. But statistics reveal that FSCs are barely reducing home fires caused by unattended cigarettes. In fact, a retired firefighter and battalion chief said one in every three house fires is still ignited by a cigarette.

When a cigarette falls in between couch cushions or between bedsheets, it doesn't really matter if the cigarette goes out a minute later. Thanks to the pesticides, ammonia, bleached paper, and now carpet glue, the lit "cherry" of a cigarette burns at up to seventeen hundred degrees Fahrenheit, so when left resting on cotton or polyester, it can smolder for hours before actually igniting into a flame. Then it can devour an entire house within minutes.

"Fire-safe" cigarettes are made with three layers of paper that require triple the glues of past cigarettes. Designed to reduce oxygen flow, the glue often puts the cigarette out too early, causing the smoker to reignite several times throughout a cigarette. This is quite ironic, because it essentially adds to the heat and the toxic release that a typical cigarette filter can't handle. In turn, it's forcing the smoker to puff harder and more frequently than they otherwise would, compounding health problems.

Smokers of the FSCs complain of migraine headaches, nausea, burning eyes and a copper metallic taste in their mouth. In addition, the carpet glue exhale, combined with carbon monoxide, can cause neurological problems for infants. Naphthalene, a core part of the "safe" cigarette, is an insecticide and a byproduct of the coal tar industry and is commonly found in mothballs. Exposure in high amounts can cause irreversible damage to the eyes and the liver and can result in malaise, confusion, anemia, convulsions and coma, according to the Environmental Protection Agency.

You can identify FSCs by the letters near the barcode on the pack or by holding the cigarettes up to the light, which makes the two bands visible. New York was the first state to require the fire-safe rings, but now nearly every state in the U.S. has jumped on the bandwagon.

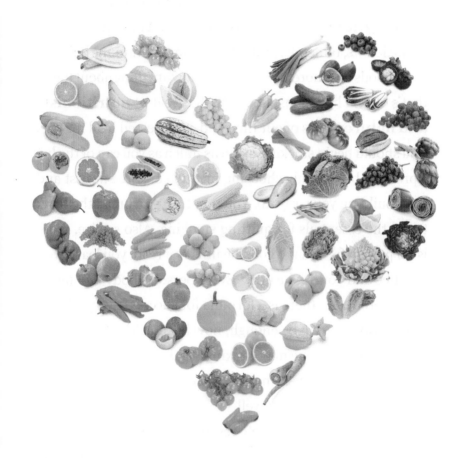

Part IV
Nutrition,
The Only Alternative

Let's get to the root of your problems. ***Disease is just a fancy word for bad nutrition.*** Your body needs antioxidants, minerals, probiotics, vitamins, immune building Superfoods and more. If you do not know anything about these, that's okay. I have consulted with the greatest **nutritionists and naturopaths** of our time and compressed it all for you. You should begin stocking up on as much as you can of the list I provide, but by only choosing just two or three at first and then building your way up. You don't have to break the bank to get the essentials for quitting smoking. Also realize, there is no perfect formula to good health. You read, you learn, you practice and you get healthy. Every person's body and needs are different, but there is a formula for success. Everything in moderation used to be enough, now it's not. The formula for success filters out the major toxins. Again, I am not inventing the wheel, or re-inventing the wheel, I'm just spinning the ones that work and work well.

Here's a short but well-researched SHOPPING LIST for remaining healthy and smoke free once you have kicked the habit in fourteen days.

Spring water has exactly what the body needs to balance your system. Spring water is vitally important to drink while you stop smoking cigarettes and after you quit. Spring water helps ensure healthy cell production.

Dark, organic chocolate is different than the cheap stuff you get in convenience store type candy bars or peanut butter cups. Organic chocolate helps promote a healthy mental condition and state of mind and acts as a natural way to replace nicotine's function. Depression!

Vitamin B complex, especially with niacin, will help balance your central nervous system, which is severely depleted due to smoking. This vitamin is sold as a complex and should be organic. Ask your naturopath or vitamin shop expert about niacin.

L-Tyrosine is an amino acid which helps fight depression, cure anxiety and chronic fatigue. Ask about branch chain amino acids at your favorite vitamin shop or online.

Mucuna (also found listed under "dopabean" and mucuna pruriens)—this helps your body in crisis situations like fight or flight, and helps with overall positive feelings and also gives you "fuel" for confidence and sex drive! Ex-smokers love this natural remedy!

Organic mushrooms (powders) are sold as a natural supplement that millions of Chinese and people of Asia and India take to build up a host of immunity to protect their bodies from viruses, diseases and infections (warning: you can NOT eat the ones that grow from the ground in your yard). Check out dried capsules or the powder form of **reishi, cordiceps, chaga and maitake and lion's mane** as part of a mushroom complex. These mushrooms build immunity and help to treat and beat certain cancers too! You won't see any advertisements on TV or hear about this on the news. They don't want you to escape your expensive habit and get healthy, but I do.

Raw vegetables

There are many myths out there about protein, especially the ones that say you have to eat meat to get enough. That's a big lie many people believe and let me tell you, if it's not organic meat, then you are consuming chemicals and that drives you to be lethargic and depressed. So then, the big question remains: What vitamins and proteins can you get from uncooked veggies that you cannot get from bread, milk, and meat? Raw vegetables have all the nutrients humans need. They also contain protein, so you don't need red meat or chicken! You can still steam some veggies like broccoli and cauliflower and get essential nutrients. Organic food and natural remedies work! Don't let anyone tell you otherwise. Check out the "Protein Myth" as dispelled by professional athlete Tim Van Orden on this YouTube clip: https://www.youtube.com/watch?v=ae-dlHOmwk4&list=PL46A830C7C79D0083

As mentioned earlier, mucuna is a natural supplement from a velvet bean that counteracts the dopamine deficiency that you have from smoking chemically treated nicotine. What happens when you don't have enough dopamine and something stressful happens? This lack of dopamine leads to anxiety, panic attacks and worst of all—lighting up a cigarette. These are safe alternatives and organic ones that are at your fingertips.

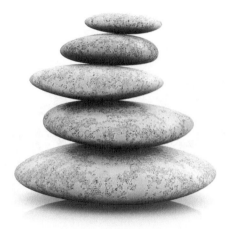

Hypnotherapy

Quitting smoking is mental and physical. After you quit—physically escape the nicotine and you supplement your heart and central nervous system with proper vitamins and nutrients—you have to address the mental aspect. What form of "coaching" is best for this mental deactivation of the cravings for a cigarette? Hypnotherapy is a good way to keep from going back to smoking. Plus, it's harmless. But you don't have to be hypnotized, just start despising cigarettes for what they did TO TRICK YOU! Then, enjoy your healthy life and you will be a nonsmoker forever!

Remember that Big Tobacco has tricked you into smoking GMO-pesticide-laden crop. Now you have the solution to detoxify yourself. What will you do to EXPEL the GMO tobacco pesticides from your body quickly, so you won't relapse and want a cigarette? Here are some answers: Milk thistle detoxifies your liver of the pesticides!! Also eat plenty of garlic in your favorite dishes, as long as you're not allergic. Check out the benefits of cinnamon also. Lastly, cabbage is fuel for boosting serotonin and dopamine.

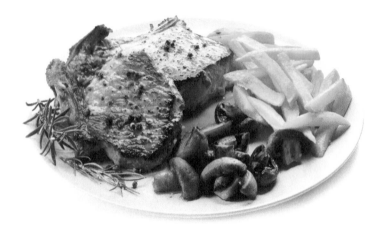

Dead food

When food is boiled, broiled, fried in oil, baked, roasted, charbroiled, microwaved or toasted, it's "dead." When food is cooked out back on the grill, especially with the lid on, it's dead, meaning the food simply loses the vitamins, enzymes, amino acids (proteins), antioxidants and all of the essential minerals that fuel every system in the human body and defend it against cancer. I'm not saying stop eating everything that's cooked, and stop cooking, I'm just pointing out which food is valuable to your body and your blood, so you can keep up and know the difference. Understand and appreciate this: When infants are fed cooked food and cooked milk, they could be getting next to zero in the nutrition department, and that can get serious rather quickly. When you get zero nutrition or even close to it, you get tired, depressed, stressed and frustrated. Imagine trying to quit cigarettes and without proper nutrition. No wonder most programs (gimmicks) fail those who try them.

Living food

Most soil in America is massively depleted of nutrients thanks to pesticides, herbicides, insecticides, pollution from factories, improper mass waste disposal from hospitals, and so on. That means that no matter how much you eat (and drink) of your favorite fruits and vegetables, if they came from toxic, polluted DEAD SOIL, then the plants did not absorb nutrients, and they can't make them up themselves. It's as simple as that. Now it's time to talk positive. Organically grown foods from rich soils are essential to your tobacco recovery and overall health. Top RAW Superfoods, like spirulina, chlorella and chia seeds, are available from the Natural News Store at affordable prices, and you can even stock up your storage of these for emergency situations.

Want the most energy possible, a super-powered immune system and fuel for your wonderful brain? Load up your pantry and fridge with some or all of the following: organic cacao powder, medicinal mushroom powders, green powders, red berry powders, spirulina, chlorella, dried superfruits, kale chips and trail mix. By stocking up with **Superfoods** you will also be preparing your home for natural disasters, emergencies and travel.

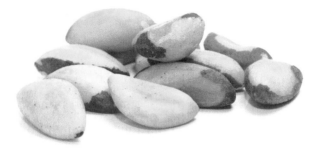

Go nuts

Raw nuts provide healthy fats that are essential to the body and lower the LDL "bad" cholesterol in the blood. Watch out though, cooked over one hundred and seventy degrees, nuts do just the opposite and cause plaque in the blood. Raw garlic provides a DNA-protecting compound. One minute of cooking, though, completely inactivates this enzyme. Grow your own garlic! It's one of the easiest perennials to grow.

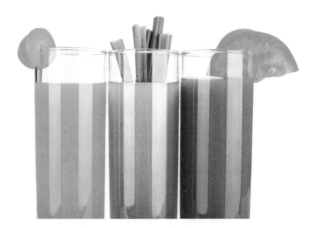

Juice it

Juice for raw fruit and vegetable juice. A fairly good juicer runs less than one hundred and fifty dollars, so now juice is easy to make at home and isn't cooked, pasteurized and then loaded with high fructose corn syrup and toxic artificial colors.

Old Salt

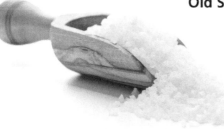

Raw salts contain trace minerals essential to good health. Table salt is typically heated to high temperatures, treated with chemicals, radiated and then bleached. This kind of salt is toxic. Raw mineral salts such as Himalayan are crucial for proper mineral balance. Also, bathing in "Dead Sea Salts" is the ultimate way to relax the muscles and detoxify your entire system! Go online. They're cheap!

Brain food

Raw cacao is brain food and contains a wealth of essential vitamins and minerals that boost the body's neurotransmitters and phytochemicals, thus activating mood-elevating emotions. Raw chia seeds (just four tablespoons) supply as much calcium as three cups of milk, as much magnesium as ten stalks of broccoli, and as much iron as one-half cup of red kidney beans.

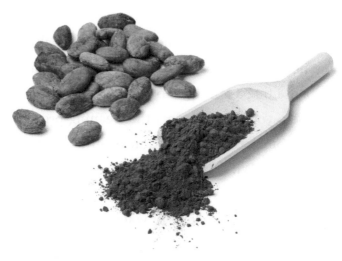

Mucuna

I cannot say enough about mucuna. The mucuna herb replaces cigarette cravings and helps kick the habit. Mucuna, also known as Velvet Bean, is capturing the interest of thousands of smokers who have the desire and the will to quit cigarettes, but can't handle the first couple of weeks (fourteen days) of rollercoasterlike mood swings and basic withdrawal symptoms. The L-dopa content of the un-processed mucuna bean powder is so powerful that doctors are also using it to 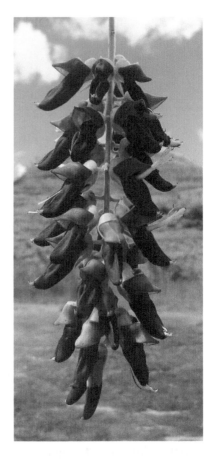 help people with Parkinson's disease restore mental clarity, and as a mood elevator.

If you can't find mucuna at a local health food or vitamin shop, and you have to order it through the mail, you may be waiting a few days to get it. When you finish reading this book, you can still start the weaning process of getting off the commercial cigarettes and shifting to organic, *without the mucuna*. When the mucuna arrives, well, then you'll have that phenomenal "boost" and take the whole routine up a notch or two! Freedom is close for you now! Feel it. Embrace it.

The wondrous Indian herb

This wondrous ayurvedic Indian herb (mucuna) is known by many names, including sea beans, buffalo beans, dopabean, pruriens, cowitch, kapikachu and atmagupta. The main medicinal benefits come from the seeds, but the pod and the roots can also be used. The velvety beans are actually drift seeds, meaning they can float away on ocean currents and re-plant themselves all over the world. Google a picture of them—they are amazing and beautiful. Remember, there is no one product or vitamin that is a cure-all, and every person's body chemistry is different than the next.

Mucuna replenishes your body

Improves sleep

Reduces body fat and cellulite

Helps with regeneration of organs (heart, kidneys, liver, lungs)

Dramatically strengthens the immune system

Improves skin appearance

Increases mood and sense of well being

Increases bone density (Very necessary after toxin overload from cigarettes, which have leached the minerals out of your bones!)

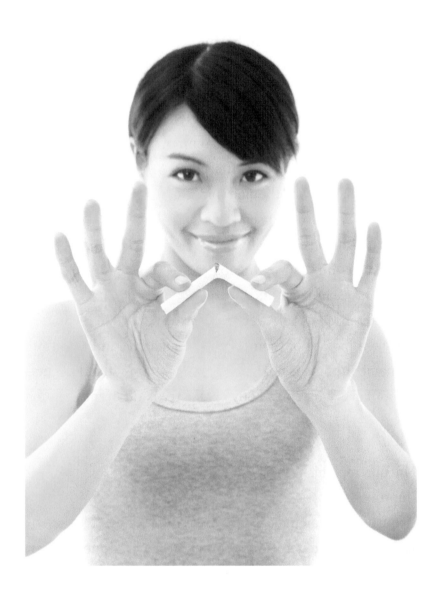

Part V
The "New You"
Does Great Things

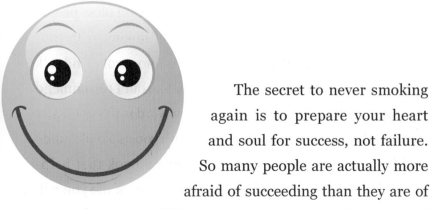

The secret to never smoking again is to prepare your heart and soul for success, not failure. So many people are actually more afraid of succeeding than they are of failing. See, success brings the weight of responsibility with it, and failure does not. But the "weight of responsibility" is all mental, because once you engage yourself in wonderful habits that give you energy and momentum, you can just put your life on cruise control and enjoy the ride. You will look back at this experience, a long time from now, and you will laugh and say to yourself, "I'm so glad I quit when I did!" For many, this program, this book, this lesson of life, it comes as a blessing in disguise. Some people stumble upon *14 & Out* when putting keywords in a search engine, like "best program in the world to stop smoking" or "stop smoking naturally." But many smokers find the *14 & Out* program because one of their friends or loved ones shared a link to one of my *YouTube* videos or to one of my blogs, or they saw one of my books of matches at a bar or restaurant that says "Quit smoking in 14 days or less!" Or, "Make this your last book of matches!"

Some people hear about *14 & Out* because Mike Adams of *Natural News* posted one of our **Skype** interviews online, or he published one of my professional articles, or better yet, one of his reporters wrote a review and covered one or more key elements of the *14 & Out* program plan. God bless people who share! Share this book after you quit smoking, with your friends, neighbors, relatives, coworkers who smoke and talk about quitting. They can also buy the video, but I recommend the paperback book because the written word is powerful and very handy. This book can be carried with you as a daily guide and inspiration. Besides *14 & Out* being a book that helps you quit smoking for good, *14 & Out* is a way of life you will always use as a strategy for overcoming adversity and staying positive.

Although my grandfather smoked himself to death when I was a little boy and I didn't get to spend much of my life with him, I feel that his soul has come back to visit me and help me reach out to smokers with a desire to quit, so they and you too can live smoke free for the rest of your lives and never suffer like he did, especially his last two years. My Grandfather Sol Gross was a good man who served in the Army and was a semi-pro golfer. He was a first generation American who moved from New York City to Richmond, Virginia, when he met and married my grandmother. He ran a ladies hat and handbag business for many years, and he was most proud to have served in the Army in World War II. He was a great father to my mother, and if he were here today to see how many people I have saved from cigarettes by the natural method, I just know he would cry with joy and hug me!

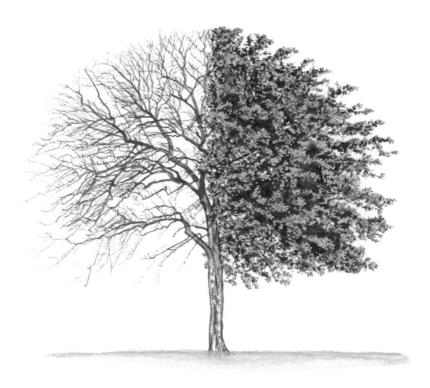

Prepare for transformation

Now imagine this: You've quit smoking and you're spending hundreds less per month. Your clothes don't smell like smoke, your breath is fresh and you've been working out and feel great. Everything is great, but then something stressful happens. Some situation arises and some friend or acquaintance standing next to you lights up a cigarette (it might even happen to be your old brand) ... and so you glance at it for a second, but then you laugh a little to yourself, and then smiling at your friend, you put up your first two fingers like you're holding one already, and you pretend to take a drag. Then you take a deep breath and exhale. ***This is your moment!*** Now you just grab a bottled water and knowing you're a nonsmoker who is never going back, you deal with reality and move forward with your healthy life. Hey, it's all mental from there.

Remember this: No one can ever choose the perfect day or time to quit smoking. I've heard friends, neighbors and relatives say every excuse in the book ... it's always, "I want to quit, but not right now though, Sean. I'm too stressed," or "Wait until I get back from vacation," or "Maybe after I get this job ...," and you get the concept. One person once told me he couldn't quit smoking because his wife would find out. I said, "What do you mean, she'll find out you quit?" He said that she didn't know he started smoking again, and when he quits, he gets really cranky and bitter, so if he quit, she would know he started up again. How ridiculous is that? If you want to fix your health and your life, just do it. Remember at the beginning of the book when I asked you to ask yourself, "Why can't I quit?" Now you know why!

In fact, most *14 & Out* ex-smokers realized there were **several reasons** they couldn't quit, and they realized it wasn't really their fault that they got dragged into smoking a pack a day or more. It's like an undertow in the ocean; if you don't learn to swim with the current, you can't learn how to escape the current. My plan has taught you how to swim with the current, using organic cigarettes for the last fourteen days, and supplementing everything you do with something organic, natural and positive. Let's bring this concept home, literally.

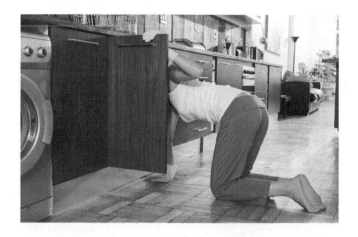

Remove the chemicals from your home

So do it now. Clean out your pantry, your refrigerator, your freezer, of all junk food, processed food, boxed meals, and microwaveable "uselessness." Toss the sugar out or give it away if you don't want to waste it. Throw out all the synthetic sugars and any food which contains them. One dose of aspartame, sucralose or sorbitol could fool your body into thinking it needs "super sweet" and you could have a chemical relapse and want to "light up." Later on, a month or two from now, you can cheat with food a little, or drinks at the bar or whatever, but never a cigarette, or you get dragged back into the pack a day undertow. Think of only holistic, wholesome living like when you were a kid. Energy and vitality brew inside you! No coughing, no shaky hands, no "quick tired" from the lack of sports or outdoor activity. No. This is really happening. You can be YOU again! Move forward and never look back. Also, keep this book with you wherever you go for the first two weeks, so you can review, recap and know what products to buy to assist your journey to freedom.

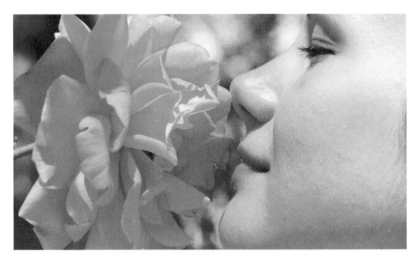

Simple pleasures return—tastebuds and sense of smell!

Guess what? In case you didn't notice, smoking kills your tastebuds and your sense of smell, almost down to nothing. When you quit smoking, these wonderful senses come back to life, and you remember how great life is with these wonderful "gifts" that reward you all day, every day. Plus, when you cut other chemical foods and "junk science" out of your daily regimen, your tastebuds can recover from the onslaught of MSG and aspartame and return to where organic food tastes amazing. You will want to cook more or just eat more raw foods, so you can slice up those vegetables and herbs and fresh fruits and taste their excellence again! By activating your sense of smell and taste to one hundred percent again, you are actually reactivating chemicals in the body that make you feel good and take more action that benefits you, like quitting cigarettes forever. I get information all the time in testimonials from ex-smokers who talk about the first few days of *14 & Out* and how they feel.

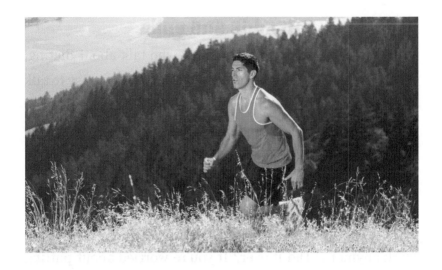

Benefits of a smoke-free life begin almost immediately:

After eight hours: Nicotine and carbon monoxide levels in the blood are halved, oxygen levels in the blood return to normal.

After twenty-four hours: Carbon monoxide is eliminated from the body, and the lungs start to clear out the buildup of tar.

After forty-eight hours: There is no nicotine left in the body. The sense of taste and smell are greatly heightened and improved!

Upon seventy-two hours: Breathing becomes easier, bronchial tubes begin to relax, energy levels increase.

From fourteen days—thereafter: Circulation improves, making walking and running a lot easier.

Source: http://www.annepenman.com/benefits

At odds and ends

How many people do you know who talk about dieting, but rarely change their health or looks? It's rather easy to talk the talk, but right now you are going to walk the walk. You see, some people bounce in and out of diets, losing ten or maybe twenty pounds, only to *put it right back on* a few months later. Some people hit that "plateau," and no matter what they do, they can't lose a pound. What about them? Where are they going wrong? Doesn't the famous "low-carb" diet work anymore? Did it ever? If you're worried about putting on weight when you quit smoking, or you want to lose weight, just follow the yellow brick road (*14 & Out*) and this will guide you to prosperity and balance. Learn what NOT to eat and drink first, and that will catapult you into wise choices.

Think for a second about people who consume "fake sugars" or artificial sweeteners. Their bodies are worn down, trying to expel toxins that are not natural to this world. These sweeteners are synthetic. But wait a second, wouldn't the FDA tell you if artificial sweeteners were toxic carcinogens? The FDA has **very few regulations** for food additives, preservatives and artificial sweeteners. Don't count on them for help in this arena.

http://www.naturalnews.com/021920_aspartame_public_safety.html

We must also ask, "What about MSG, monosodium glutamate, and its addictive power?" Do any doctors, pharmacists, cancer specialists or TV talk shows mention how artificial sweeteners and MSG are addictive and actually make you FAT? Oh, you didn't know? ***Artificial Sweetener Disease*** (ASD) is sweeping the country. MSG is in hundreds of foods, yet monosodium glutamate is a leading cause of migraine headaches and central nervous system imbalance. Your job is to filter it out of your intake. Food "drugs" can make you relapse and want to smoke again. What artificial sweeteners cause the most damage to your body, blood and organs? *Aspartame, sorbitol, saccharine* and *sucralose* are the biggest culprits. Are they part of your daily routine? Check your soda, coffee and tea. **Check your gum, mints and candy.**

http://www.naturalnews.com/034378_artificial_ sweetener_disease_ASD_aspartame.html

Check your **toothpaste and mouthwash.** Throw away your cough syrups and antacids. Toxic sweeteners show up in most food labeled "light," "zero" or "fat free."

You could easily replace sugar with a safe, natural low-cal or zero-cal sweetener like *xylitol* or *Stevia*. Also, organic honey is a great sweetener, just consume in moderation!

This recognition and filtering of food "toxins" is very important if you are concerned about putting on weight when quitting smoking. You body is craving nutrients and should be rewarded with whole foods that replenish your system, not drive it back to the state it was in before you quit.

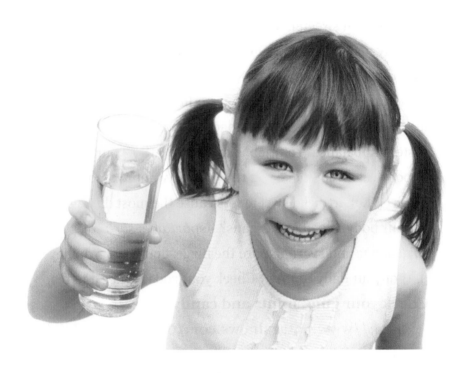

Drug Water

Did you know that U.S. water fluoridation began in 1945 and continues today, despite the fact that the FDA has never approved it. There's nothing worse than drinking water to hydrate yourself, only to be secretly dehydrating yourself, leaching calcium and magnesium from your bones, and actually assisting the "aging" process. Anyone trying to stop smoking needs spring water, or at least water that has been through a process called reverse osmosis, which removes harmful metals like aluminum and takes out the fluoride, bleaches and even medications that flow through the water of the municipal taps nearly everywhere. Remember, spring water is the absolute best. Don't fall for the great FLUORIDE HOAX when they say it's good for your teeth. It is not. There is extensive research. Check it out on YouTube, Natural

News, and InfoWars.com, where alternative news tells it like it really is. Think fluoride evaporates from water? Fluoride does not evaporate from water left sitting out. Also, boiling or freezing won't help at all, and basic filters like Brita do not remove it. Reverse osmosis does remove it, and natural spring water does not contain it.

http://www.infowars.com/some-non-organic-foods-contain-upwards-of-180-times-the-fluoride-level-of-tap-water-says-expert/

"Fluoridigate"—Watch the documentary! https://www.youtube.com/watch?v=LrWFnGpX9wY

Fight water fluoridation in your city!

http://www.naturalnews.com/036084_water_fluoridation_protests_activism.html

Drink spring water or water that has been through reverse osmosis!

Fluoridated water is an American tragedy

Fluoride has never received FDA approval and does not meet "requirements of safety and effectiveness." The FDA states that fluoride is a prescription drug. Because this "drug" is put in municipal water, there is absolutely no control over individual dosage. Imagine, if you will, someone trying to quit a chemical addiction when there's one in the tap water!

http://blogs.naturalnews.com/fluoridated-water-and-brain-performance-linked/

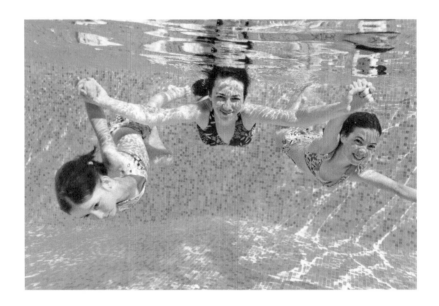

This is why 14 & Out is unique. I point out all the major factors blocking the path to freedom, and all you have to do is follow the "yellow brick road."

For finding natural springs (spring water coming out of the rocks pure as possible) go to findaspring.com, and you may just need to gather up some five gallon water jugs and go on a road trip! Keep life simple, clean and positive. Your life is an adventure to be enjoyed, not an addiction to Big Tobacco. Find clean, clear, perfect water and find your "perfect" day.

http://www.findaspring.com/

Big Tobacco's Seventy-five-Year Brainwash

For over seventy-five years, cigarettes have been pushed on the American masses through advertisements on television, radio, in magazines and on billboards, but few people realize that the initial "evil seeds of thought" were planted in the 1930s, when Camel convinced smokers that cigarettes *aid in digestion,* beginning and perpetuating the myth. The year was 1936, and the horribly misleading Camel advertisement featured doctors, yes I said doctors, who recommended smoking at least one cigarette between each course of your Thanksgiving dinner "for digestion's sake." The ad was FDA approved and appeared in *Life* magazine, and was intended to infuse a psychological addiction that convinced smokers they could build up a sense of "digestive well-being." Camel used convincing tag lines saying they "Never tire the taste or get on the nerves," and (Camels) "Speed up the flow of digestive fluids," "Increase alkalinity," and "Help your digestion to run smoothly," and of course, "Good food and tobacco go together naturally!"

Do you know that the U.S., Japan and China alone make up over three-fourths of the world's smokers? It's true. All over the world, children and teens still recognize the **Marlboro Man** and **Joe Camel** as being "cool," and women have consistently been a target (target market) for cigarette advertising, pushing the tall and slim look. The problem is that even if you're tall and slim, you still get the same kind of cancer.

Marlboro is "The King," the number one selling premium brand cigarette in the world, because of the highest potency rating of their "custom made" **nicotine delivery device**. Make no mistake about it. The other KINGS of the industry are all in on the evil trick also, including *Winston, Lucky Strike, Kool, Parliament, Pall Mall, Camel and Newport,* and of course, the *menthols.* The scam to hook smokers by using ammonia to strengthen the nicotine addiction WORKS, and the four thousand plus chemicals in commercial cigarettes are no joke, leading the smoker right off the cliff, where they feel like their only way out of feeling awful is to light up. http://www.naturalnews.com/037232_Mucuna_cigarette_cravings_kick_the_habit.html#ixzz2e35VpzJb

http://www.the-top-tens.com/lists/top-ten-cigarette-brands.asp

The recent "warning ads" about the effects of smoking are not educational, nor do they help smokers understand strategies for cessation at all.

Do you remember the campaign of commercials that show people suffering from diseases and disorders caused by smoking? Guess what, a U.S. appeals court in Washington D.C. recently blocked the requirement that tobacco companies would have to begin putting large graphic health warnings on the cigarette packages! R.J. Reynolds leads the way again for Big Tobacco and has blocked the FDA mandate. How convenient!

Interview with the Health Ranger

Once in a while, life grants us a phenomenal opportunity. When you get to speak with someone about your passion, whether it be art, music, books, health or just hobbies, and that person has **millions of health enthusiasts** who listen to/follow his/her advice, well, you make the most of it! I was able to talk to Mike Adams about the strategies that work for *14 & Out*, how I came up with the whole program and its name, and you may be surprised how deep my passion and this project really runs!

Mike Adams says that, "Despite its stated mission, 'to promote the art and science of medicine and the betterment of public health,' the *American Medical Association* (AMA) has taken *many missteps* in protecting the health of the American people. One of the most striking examples is the AMA's long-term relationship with the tobacco industry. Camel ran ads in the 1930s where doctors told you all about their favorite brands they smoke!

http://www.naturalnews.com/021949_Big_Tobacco_the_AMA. html#ixzz2bIxJI1ez

This is straight from the Health Ranger's article: "The *Journal of the American Medical Association* (JAMA) published its first cigarette advertisement in 1933, stating that it had done so only 'after careful consideration of the extent to which cigarettes were used by physicians in practice.' " These advertisements continued for twenty years. The same year, **Chesterfield** began running ads in the *New York State Journal of Medicine*, with the claim that its cigarettes were "Just as pure as the water you drink ... and practically untouched by human hands."

I'm telling you right now, watch out who you trust with your health and welfare. There have been over one hundred years of corruption in the USA with regards to "Big Pharma," better known as Western Medicine. Today's broken medical system has the same exact core flaw as the *Flexner Report* from **one hundred years ago**, which offered severely limited choices and stifled competition, which is ultimately regulated and controlled by state governments, *Big Pharma* and the AMA (*American Medical Association*). The ultimate result of this relentless **campaign of misinformation** and these suppressed alternative therapies is decreased access to quality medical care.

Also, for most Americans, the word *conspiracy* means having a paranoid delusion about the government having complete control over a situation, but as research reveals for *more than one hundred years*, the **Flexner Report of 1910** was the beginning of a conspiracy (yes, I said it) to limit and eventually eliminate competition from non-drug, non-patentable cancer therapies and cures. Plus, pro-establishment organizations like the *American Cancer Society* (ACS), the *National Cancer Institute* (NCI), and the *Diabetes Foundation* control the news and local medical boards to the degree that the old theory of "medical conspiracy" has become a reality, offering **only toxic therapies** for cancer that add up to billions in profits for the "organized" medical industry.

http://www.healingcancernaturally.com/medical-history.html

25 Amazing (and Disturbing) Facts about the Hidden History of Medicine

Download the free report:

http://www.naturalnews.com/RR-25-Amazing-Facts-About-Hidden-History-Medicine.html

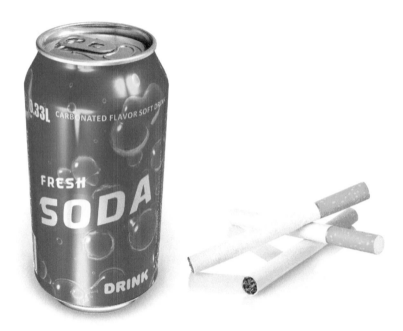

Big Question: Cigarettes or Diet Soda— Which is Worse?

Most people who smoke a pack a day of cigarettes know they are treading on thin ice regarding their health, but how many people realize that drinking thirty or more ounces of diet soda each day could prove to be more lethal than a pack of cigarettes? And how can diet soda be worse than regular soda? Even though there are over four thousand chemicals in one commercial cigarette, the leading chemical in diet soda may actually be breeding more cancer cells in human beings, and thus leading to malignant tumors sooner in life, according to recent research. http://naturalsociety.com

Could cancer be the end result of depression? Killing brain neurons and expediting cell death may be killing people faster than lung cancer, and chronic depression is fuel for overwhelming cell mutation and the taking over of organs by mutagenic warped cells, also known as blood cancer.

http://www.holisticmed.com/aspartame/

People who smoke cigarettes are locked into a vicious cycle of boosting their confidence and dopamine levels with a highly addictive drug, nicotine. The cigarette hangover, which begins with **smoking four thousand chemicals** and then waiting for the nicotine to subside, is just the beginning of lung cancer and the mutation of cells.

Cancer thrives in an acidic body where the cells are deprived of oxygen and nutrients. Yet, *even worse* than cigarettes are artificial sweeteners, which fool the body into ingesting them, as if they are food, and polluting the cleansing organs with mutagens. Some research shows the body never excretes all of the aspartame, *sorbitol, sucralose* or *saccharine*. When a human consumes *Equal, Splenda, Nutrasweet, Sweet'N Low, etc.*, their cleansing organs, like the **liver, kidneys** and **pancreas**, are overworking and malnourished. You cannot live without these organs. Aspartame is a GMO, so the blood is infected with synthetic carcinogens (which it does not release properly, if ever) which cause **central nervous system (CNS) disorders** and make you hungrier! That's right, synthetic sugars drive hunger and actually make most people put on weight. How ironic, right? Can you believe they put vitamins in synthetic, toxic products to trick you into using them? Which ones? Here's a source:

http://www.naturalnews.com/033914_Splenda_Essentials_ sweetener.html

http://www.naturalnews.com/039857_cancer_cigarettes_diet_ soda.html

It is proven that obesity is a driving force of cancer, so whether you consume excess sugar or artificial sweeteners, you are feeding the *same destructive forces* in your body, in your cells, **changing your DNA**, and the long-term effects have "no cure." So, when it all boils down to it, drinking three or four diet sodas per day is more dangerous than smoking a pack of cigarettes, about twenty cigarettes, in one day. Although diet sodas contain less chemicals than cigarettes, these specific "diet" chemicals are choking cells and mutating DNA at a higher rate, leading to chronic disorders of the digestive track, breakdown of the CNS and ultimately lead to the development of cancerous tumors. It is "programmed cell death" and your **mitochondria** are basically suffocating. If you combine toxic food and toxic medications prescribed by *Western doctors* (MDs), the addictions being "programmed in" are like programming an early death. http://www.zenantidiet.com/

Currently, there exists no prescription drug, and there will never be one, which cures the problems that artificial sweeteners create. Over seventy percent of reported cases of **fibromyalgia, chronic depression, IBS** and **acid reflux** are caused by consuming chemical agents that have been approved by the FDA. The good news is that there are **natural cures** for both diet soda addiction and cigarette addiction. They are called Superfoods and this has been studied in great depth and detail. http://www.naturalnews. com/039534_superfoods_healing_organic.html

Top Superfoods

Do you want the very best nutrition, USDA-approved organic, Superfoods, healthy storable food and safe natural remedies? Check out the Natural News Store and read Mike Adams's reviews and recommendations. Also read the "Top 10 Superfoods" the Health Ranger eats every day. http://www.naturalnews.com. The Health Ranger Mike Adams is an honest man who does his best to empower hundreds of thousands of people every day. His advice is based on in-depth research and is a phenomenal path to ideal health. http://www.naturalnews.com/040801_superfoods_disease_prevention_heart_health.html

Sources for this section of research include:
http://www.holisticmed.com/aspartame/
http://naturalsociety.com

More Superfood sources:
http://www.zenantidiet.com/
http://www.cancerresearchuk.org
http://store.naturalnews.com/Superfoods_c_4.html

Nutrition kicks the cigarette fix!

http://www.naturalnews.com/041536_nutrition_cigarettes_addiction.html

The finish line

You have just made one of the best choices of your lifetime by making the decision to stop smoking and by choosing *14 & Out* to help you accomplish this goal. Your decision will not only make your life better, but it will also improve the lives of those around you. You already have the drive to quit, and with *14 & Out*, now you have the tools and the knowledge to never light up a cigarette again for as long as you live. This natural process of quitting smoking is the best, most realistic approach, and several hundred testimonials have poured in to confirm that the answer is in your hands right now! I thank my grandfather in Heaven for the ability and motivation to communicate his message to the thousands of people who want their healthy life back, the one they had before they picked up that first cancer stick. Move forward and begin anew now. *14 & Out* welcomes you to the nonsmoker family.

The "Stop Smoking King" is on YouTube

There is a video clip posted from the class on *YouTube* (Thousands of views) https://www.youtube.com/watch?v=Zo6vwNgzfVQ

Trivial "Pursuit" *14 & Out* style

You've played *20 Questions* before, but did it change your life?! These points are taken from the twenty- question pop quiz given in the *14 & Out* classroom. All questions are posed, guesses are made, and then answers are revealed. You can take the quiz too and even get the sources, website links and video clips for the answers. Everything is at your fingertips. Take your best guesses now, then log on and get the answers to the quiz, or just finish reading the book and you will know!

Let's play "20 Questions" and see how much you learned:

1. Can you name five ingredients in a cigarette?

2. Why are cigarettes white?

3. Why are cigarettes so addicting?

4. How does the tobacco plant and seeds contain poison in the fields of America?

5. Why does it take up to fifteen years for a cigarette filter to disintegrate?

6. Why do cigarettes burn so hot, so evenly, and never go out in heavy wind?

7. What effect do all of the chemicals have on your body?

8. Why do the pills, the patch and nicotine gum fail so many?

9. What government agencies regulate the potency of nicotine?

10. Other than nicotine, what else is there that you're addicted to?

11. Is your breathing pattern better when smoking?

12. Do you have a hand-to-mouth habit?

13. Is smoking a form of meditation?

14. Why do most smokers enjoy a cigarette after meals?

15. Is there any such thing as organic tobacco?

16. What is the art of breathing?

17. Why do people often put on weight after they quit?

18. How can you learn to hate cigarettes if you like them now?

19. How will you deal with the urge and with stress?

20. What's the main reason the pills don't work, but makes things worse?

Answers to
Twenty Questions
"that will make you quit smoking."

http://www.naturalnews.com/040967_stop_smoking_
cigarette_addiction_14andOut.html#ixzz2bIq4PLG7.html

Acknowledgments

As the author, creator and teacher of *14 & Out*, naturally I would first like to thank every student who has taken my class and given themselves the opportunity to stop smoking and given me the opportunity to share my method with them. Many of the people who quit smoking using my natural method have written testimonials and kind words about their healthy life without cigarettes, and there is no greater reward to me than knowing they have quit smoking.

Many thanks go out to Mike Adams, the Health Ranger and Editor of Natural News, for whom I have been writing for two years, and who has inspired me, coached me, given me wonderful projects to tackle, has published over one hundred and fifty of my articles and who has promoted the *14 & Out* instructional video, which was the "prelude" to the book. Mike Adams's relentless pursuit of truth with regards to health freedom and natural remedies from around the world and his authenticity in journalism and reporting, have given new height, depth and expertise to my career as a writer.

Much of the research for this book has been drawn from scientific studies done by major universities in the United States, the United Kingdom and in Canada, including professional articles, interviews and books based on cigarettes and cancer research done at the University of Georgia, Johns Hopkins University, Oregon Health & Science University, Ontario Institute for Cancer Research and Bath University in the United Kingdom.

Also, I am very grateful to know David Wolfe, world famous nutritionist and world traveler, who has spoken with me personally about the cigarette addiction and the ability of proper nutrition to kill the cravings of nicotine, and all those natural remedies that replenish damaged digestive and breathing systems to enable "ex-smokers" to stay smoke free for life. His knowledge of Superfoods and alkalizing of the body has helped me develop the third phase of *14 & Out*, which makes it unique and more powerful than any other smoking cessation program in the world.

I would like to thank my fiancée, Kristine, for "opening the window" to my ultimate dream, writing for a living. Thanks also to my sisters Sandy and Stacy, a lawyer and a newspaper reporter, respectively, for their continued support and faith in me. Thank you to my father for your words of inspiration too!

Lastly and mostly, I must thank my mother, Sheila Gross Minnich, who has assisted me with her enthusiasm, ideas, knowledge, inspiration, editing, and who blessed me with my writing ability by giving birth to me, making sure I survived "growing up" and who made sure I went to college and learned my ABCs.

Testimonials

Please note: The following are all e-mails I have personally received within the last eighteen months. Full names have been shortened for privacy purposes:

"Sean, I AM doing very well. I am also no longer a smoker!! I took an evening to myself to watch the video and go over the packet. I had one cigarette after the video because my boyfriend upset me. It was the worst and last cigarette I will ever smoke! I taped a few of the handouts to my bathroom mirror to keep me motivated to quit. The picture of the lungs really puts things into perspective.. The first 3-4 days, I was one irritable young lady! But I got through it and will NEVER go back. I have been a nonsmoker for 6 weeks now and I feel great. I now go to the gym regularly and eat healthier. Your video changed my life! I am trying to help other people quit and change their lives as well. Three positive things about *14 & Out*: 1) This program was made from the heart to help others change their lives for the better. 2) If you believe in yourself you can become a nonsmoker with this program! 3) *14 & Out* changed my life completely and I've never been so happy and stress free. I cannot thank you enough Sean, you have changed my life forever. I appreciate what you do every day for others, it melts my heart."

—Erica"

"I tried e-cigs and the patch and kept going back to smoking. Give this a shot! I smoked a pack a day for 15 years and quit after this."

—Anonymous

"We have purchased and watched your *14 & Out* video, and purchased the mucuna supplement. Love your video, SO informative! Just want to be done with the whole cigarette thing. (Your video grossed me out—I can't believe we put that "nasty" in our bodies)— Thank you for your time in advance,

—Scott & Jennifer"

"I learned more in 60 minutes than I ever thought I would. It's easy to see how much hard work and careful consideration went into this program."

—Dr. B. Rose; Naturopath/Orthomolecular Medicine

"Hey Sean! My name is Lori. I've tried every smoking cessation program probably known to man and still haven't quit, unfortunately. Mike Adams recommended it so I tried it. I will say that it's the most informative program I've seen yet, and since about April I've been off the pesticide ridden tobacco. To me it's a great accomplishment, and since the natural stuff is an eye-opener to what the yucky stuff really is, I think it won't be long now. Yours is the best program hands down. I've been informing others on the truth you provide as well ... Thank you so much,

—Lori"

"Thank you for helping me free myself from that awful habit!

—Donna M: 35 year smoker"

"It has been around 4 or 5 months since I quit tobacco. I never even think about it anymore. I will never EVER, EVER go back to tobacco. The toxic tobacco cancer industry has lost a customer for life, and I say that with great delight! If someone had told me 6 months ago how easy it really is to quit once you know the dopamine and nicotine connection, I would have thought they were messing with me. But it so true, your program made it unbelievably easy, and I am so thankful for your program and hope you become rich from your program, which helps people, instead of the other side that gets rich off people's misery. I can't thank you enough, keep up the great work, thanks again!

—Robbie"

"I quit 4 days after starting *14 & Out*! Once you explained to me about my breathing habit and about ammonia and pesticide in the tobacco, I followed everything else you said to do, including the supplements and I don't even have cravings anymore!!! Thank you.

—Mike G."

"I kept saying to myself that its never a good time to quit, because I'm always stressed and I didn't want to be more stressed, but *14 & Out* gave me insight into my problem and advice on nutrition AND how to stay positive the whole time.

I watched the video and did the hands on activities. That's what got me to quit! I highly recommend this program, even if you're stressed out. Any smokers out there, if you're saying 'It's not a good time to quit, well, hey, it's NEVER a good time to die! Check out *14 & Out*, this guy will show you why you haven't quit yet, and you'll finally know how to!"

—Allen C., Athens, GA

"Thanks to *14 & Out*, I have switched to organic tobacco and only smoke a few self-rolled cigarettes a day. I feel one hundred percent better. The genius of your course is what made me throw away my store bought ones. You were right, the chemicals just wore me down and made me crave more. You were right about the supplements too. I bought some vitamin B complex and the mucuna helped very much! Keep up the great work Sean." —CJM

"Dear Sean, yes, I did watch your video and I did most of the hands on activities. I grew up on a farm so I was already familiar with some of the things on there such as ammonia and pesticides. I tried mucuna extract and plan on adding L-tyrosine. I did quit with the help of the mucuna extract and your hand's on activities! There are several things that stood out in your program. Some of the things I learned were the supplementation of vitamins and minerals along with the breathing techniques and how to simulate your smoking habits by taking breaks and using your hand habits. Thanks for your response to me after my purchase of your program. It is much appreciated and doesn't happen with any other programs." —T.M.

"Hi, I'm doing great!!! Thank you. Yes I have quit smoking and feel pretty darn good about it! I did watch the whole video, but did not do the hands on activities. I had already started a nutritional program including juicing and trying to go 100% organic. The best thing about *14 & Out* was the knowledge it provided me with. That in turn completely changed my mind on how I felt about smoking and gave me the power to quit. Thanks a million!"

—Cathy

"Now smokers don't have to be afraid of becoming a nervous, disgruntled wreck when they stop smoking. Great program and strategies shared very well." —Dr. D. Roebuck.

"I smoked a pack a day for twenty years, now I've quit for good. My business is doing better and so am I, thanks to *14 & Out*."

—P. Gordon

"I've been waiting for someone to answer all of my questions about smoking. Thank you so much!"

—DiFlorio

"Thank you for the inspiration, strategies, and momentum you create. It's like I have a new chance at life."

—Purcell

REFERENCE GUIDE

My research

Professional articles, interviews and books based on cigarettes and cancer research were studied and analyzed to create my program and make it authentic. Thank you to the universities across the globe that do REAL research and don't lie about the results. My master's degree afforded me the ability to sift through all the good, the bad and the ugly, and invent and design this natural program. I am forever grateful for your efforts and years of research:

The University of Georgia, Athens, GA., USA
Johns Hopkins University, USA
Oregon Health & Science University, USA
Bath University, UK—special thanks for the reports!
Ontario Institute for Cancer Research, Canada

Huge thanks to Mike Adams and S.D. Wells for the "Amazing Facts about the Hidden History of Medicine," an investigative report. Get the free download! It's amazing. There are two series of twenty-five professional articles with solid sources available as a safe PDF download from the Health Ranger:

http://www.naturalnews.com/RR-25-Amazing-Facts-About-Hidden-History-Medicine.html

Special thanks to The University of Georgia for my seven years of research and enlightenment in Journalism, Education and Mass Communication.

Supporting research and websites for further study: University of Georgia; cancer research links:

http://cancercenter.uga.edu/people/mpierce.html

http://cancercenter.uga.edu/expertise/prevention.html

My appearances (live broadcast sessions) on Blog Talk Radio out of New York:

http://www.blogtalkradio.com/johnwallace/2013/05/29/the-week-in-review

14 & Out; Skype interview with Health Ranger Mike Adams:

http://tv.naturalnews.com/v.asp?v=3C93710BC1C921A18E787CEC4 45DA436

Medical information from nurses and physicians:

http://www.appliedradiology.com/

http://www.radiologyassistant.nl/en/p42459cff38f02

http://www.medhelp.org/posts/Asthma-and-Allergy/Long-term-exposure-to-Fiberglass-Insulation/show/921978

http://www.asbestos.com/asbestos/smoking/

http://www.clevelandclinicmeded.com/

http://www.naturalnews.com/035766_cigarettes_glass_fibers_lung_damage.html#ixzz2BkvUcTv3

http://naturaltreatmentsforcancer.blogspot.com/

Fibrous Glass and Cancer:

http://www.ncbi.nlm.nih.gov/pubmed/7810554

http://www.ncbi.nlm.nih.gov/pubmed/10380162

http://cebp.aacrjournals.org/content/9/9/977.full

Natural News store and remedy connections:

http://store.naturalnews.com/

http://store.naturalnews.com/Detox-Support_c_12.html

http://store.naturalnews.com/Superfoods_c_4.html

Mucuna effect on free radicals:

http://www.ncbi.nlm.nih.gov/

pubmed/12237810?dopt=Abstract

"Cigarettes with defective filters marketed for 40 years: What Philip Morris never told smokers"

http://www.ncbi.nlm.nih.gov/pmc/articles/PMC1766058/

Nutrition Experts:

http://www.davidwolfe.com/

http://www.atsjournals.org/journal/ajrccm

http://www.ucomparehealthcare.com/drs/kenneth_kochler/

David Wolfe speaking about the safety of the natural herb mucuna:

https://www.youtube.com/watch?v=wIVwil2TN8Y

David Wolfe speaking regarding nervous system rejuvenation:

https://www.youtube.com/watch?v=3ryAIUhhxvs

Medical and science key term search methods:

http://science.naturalnews.com/

http://www.greenmedinfo.com/

Nutrition and herbal remedy references/links:

http://www.naturalnews.com/037232_Mucuna_cigarette_cravings_kick_the_habit.html

World's #1 Healing Secrets Newsletter and source for ordering mucuna:

http://www.raysahelian.com/mucunapruriens.html

Order Mucuna online (the amazing herbal adaptagen)

http://herbal-powers.com/herbal_powers_osc/index.php?cPath=72_76

http://www.secrets-of-longevity-in-humans.com/mucuna-pruriens.html

http://www.naturalnews.com/037232_Mucuna_cigarette_cravings_kick_the_habit.html#ixzz2BkwyobRS

14 & Out preview of video download by Mike Adams, the Health Ranger:

http://premium.naturalnews.tv/*14 & Out__*TV.htm

"Big Tobacco" on the record:
Blue Cross beats Big Tobacco in court!

http://www.rkmc.com/firm/selected-matters/minnesota-tobacco-litigation

http://www.mnwelldir.org/docs/history/quackery.htm

Why is arsenic in cigarettes?

http://www.knowswhy.com/why-is-arsenic-in-cigarettes/

"The Horrors of Chantix and Zyban" – a Natural News exclusive report:

http://www.naturalnews.com/033621_Chantix_Zyban.html

"The Dark Side of Smoking — What Big Tobacco Does NOT Want You To Know"

http://www.naturalnews.com/034374_smoking_Big_Tobacco_
addictions.html#ixzz2Bkwij8rB

Supporting blogs and links for healthy living:

http://*14 & Out*.blogspot.com/

http://stopsmokingking.wordpress.com/

http://*14 & Out*.wordpress.com/

http://naturalnewsradar.wordpress.com/

http://donteatcancer.blog.com/

http://www.findaspring.com/

Link to my other book "Don't Eat Cancer" as PDF download:
http://programs.webseed.com/Dont_Eat_Cancer__TV.htm

Search these books, poetry and concepts for helpful and insightful information

Gary Snyder: Rip Rap Poems (it's time to relax and celebrate your accomplishment)

http://www.poetryoutloud.org/poem/176577

Zen Poetry (get in the mood to appreciate the yin of your yang)

Breathing Techniques

Dr. Lorraine Day http://www.drday.com/

Medicinal Mushrooms http://www.medicalmushrooms.net/

Findaspring.com: (where you can find spring water from the ground nearest you and bottle it!)

Matrixtransformation.com

Guraw.com

PuritansPride.com

TheVitaminShoppe.com

Blessedherbs.com—colon cleansers

drnatura.com/Colon-Cleanse

herbdoc.com/kidney cleanse

SacredChocolate.com—David Wolfe—world famous nutritionist/traveler/speaker

Special reminder about supplements:

Remember, all supplements are not for everyone. I am not a doctor. Consult your favorite Naturopathic Physician* or Nutritional Specialists and do more research online or at your local library. Find a **Naturopath Doctor** near you.

http://www.naturopathic.org/AF_MemberDirectory.asp?version=2

Check out Mike Adams, the Health Ranger, on Natural News:

http://www.naturalnews.com/Index-Books.html

http://www.naturalnews.com/Index-Infographics.html

Listen to Natural News Radio 24/7/365!

http://radio.naturalnews.com/

14 & Out!
The Most Comprehensive
Smoking Cessation Program Ever!

Where there is a will, there is a way.

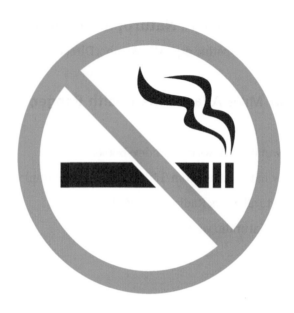

"We all live with myths that undermine our capacity to fight cancer. For example, many of us are convinced that it is primarily linked to our genetic make up, rather than our lifestyle. When we look at the research, however, we can see that the opposite is true."

—Dr David Serran-Schreiber